First Edition
Genuine Autographed Collectible

_____   _____

Do you want me to sign it in ink or in lipstick?

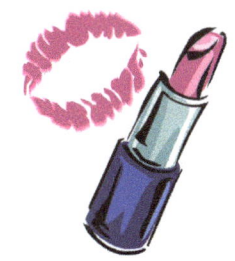

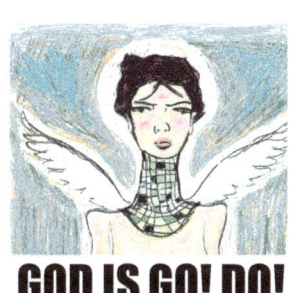

Date:

To:

From:

Message:

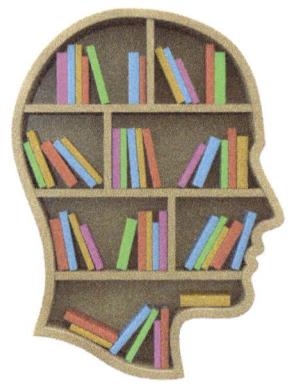

What Do Books Do?

BOOKS ARE POWERFUL!

Books Educate!
Books Enlighten!
Books Empower!
Books Entertain!
Books Emancipate!
Books Spring Eternal!
Books Drive Exploration!
Books Spark Evolution!
Books Ignite Revolution!

Sharon Esther Lampert

BooksArePowerful.com

"Bold! Brilliant! Brava!"

THE BOOK THAT WROTE ITSELF!
January 31, 2021, 1 a.m. - 10 a.m.

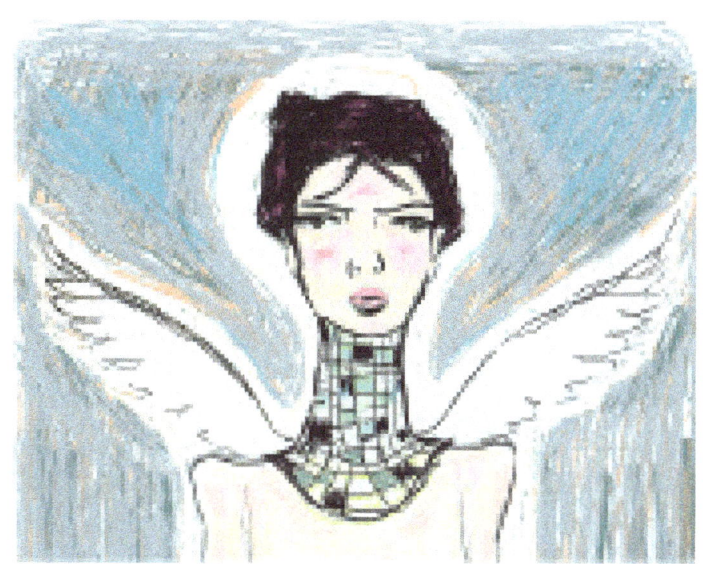

Who Knew God Was Such a Chatterbox?

Rave Book Reviews!

"For Wisdom Worshippers—The Light at the End of the Tunnel!" —Robert Cohen

"God Is Alive and Well! She Has a New Prophetess!" —Karen Moss

"God Is the Narrator. We Will Listen and Obey!" —Stephanie Marcus

"God Is a She. I Always Knew That in My Heart!" — Christopher Dunn

God, Divinity, Religion, Spirituality, Theology, Psychology, Genius, Sharon Esther Lampert

Who Knew God Was Such a Chatterbox

©2023 ©2022 First Edition by Sharon Esther Lampert. All Rights Reserved.
No part of this book may be used or reproduced in any manner whatsoever without written permission except in the case of brief quotations embodied in critical articles and reviews.

KADIMAH PRESS books may be purchased for education, business, or sales promotional use.

KADIMAH PRESS Gifts of Genius

ISBN Hardcover: 978-1-885872 - 33-3
ISBN Paperback: 978-1-885872 - 34-0
ISBN E-Book: 978-1-885872 - 36-4
Library of Congress Catalog Card Number: 2021902457

Author Contact Information
GodIsGoDo.com
Prophet@GodIsGoDo.com
Sharon@PhilosopherQueen.com
FANS@PhilosopherQueen.com
DearGod@PhilosopherQueen.com

Cover and Interior Book Design:
Creative Genius Sharon Esther Lampert
Editor: Dave Segal

Publisher: PalmBeachBookPublisher.com
Phone: 917-767-5843
Email: Sharon@PalmBeachBookPublisher.com

To Order Book:
Ingram, 1 Ingram Blvd. La Vergne, TN 37086-3629
Phone: 615-793-5000
Fax orders: 615-287-6990

First Edition
Manufactured in the United States of America

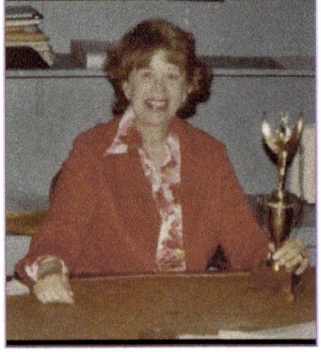

Age 9
"THE QUEEN HAS ARRIVED!
My daughter is a poet, philosopher, and teacher.
She is the Princess & the Pea!
BEAUTY & BRAINS!"
MOMMY, XOXO

MOMMY
LOVE OF MY LIFETIME!
Knew Who I Was From The
INSIDE OUT!

Sharon Esther Lampert

"A Study in Imagination, Creativity, and Genius!"
—Eve Paikoff, Ardent Fan

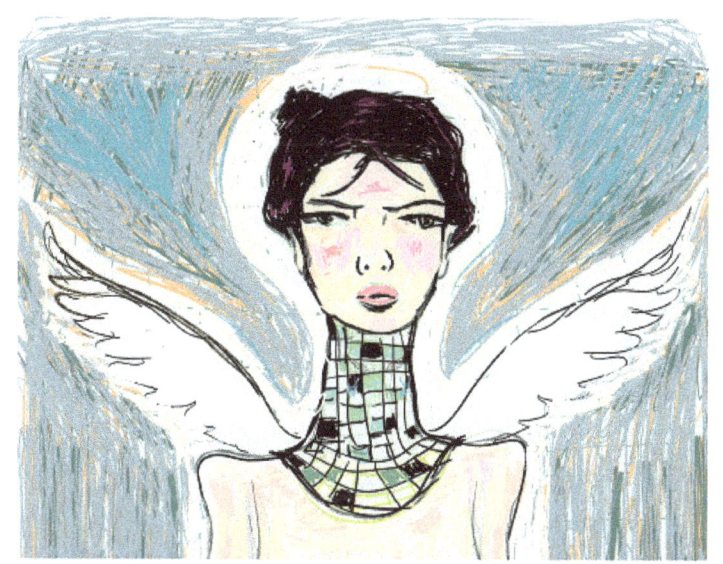

Who Knew God Was Such a Chatterbox?

God Talks to Me
A *Working* Definition of God

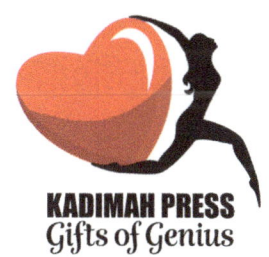

KADIMAH PRESS
Gifts of Genius

NYU AWARD for "Multi-Interdisciplinary Studies"
(YOUTUBE video)

SHARON ESTHER LAMPERT

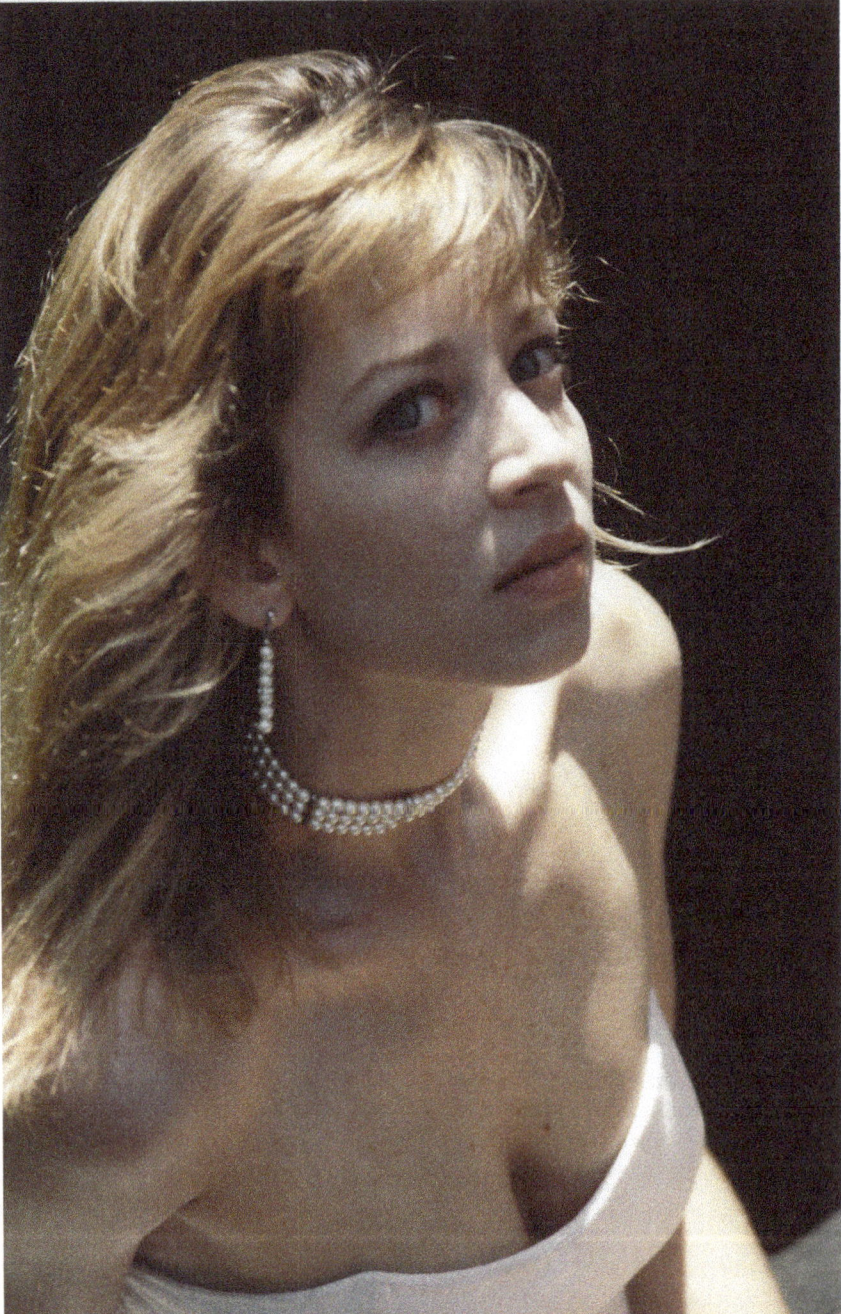

- Prodigy
- Poet
- Prophet
- Philosopher
- Peacemaker
- Paladin of Education
- **PHOTON SUPERHERO**
- Princess **KADIMAH**
- Princess & Pea
- Performer: Vocalist
- Player: Jock NYU Varsity B-Ball
- President
- Publisher
- Producer
- Psychobiologist: Rockefeller University Paper
- Piano-Playing Cat
- Phoenix
- PINUP

WEBSITES:
- SharonEstherLampert.com
- WorldFamousPoems.com
- PoetryJewels.com
- PhilosopherQueen.com
- GodIsGoDo.com
- Schmaltzy.com
- TrueLoveBurnsEternal.com
- SillyLittleBoys.com
- WinAtThin.com
- WritersRunTheWorld.com
- PalmBeachBookPublisher.com
- BooksArePowerful.com
- HappyGrandparenting.com
- WomenHaveAllThePower.com

EDUCATION:
- Smartgrades.com
- PhotonSuperHero.com
- EveryDayAnEasyA.com
- BooksNotBombs.com

Dedication

To My Gift The Creative Apparatus
Unleash The Creator The God Within

Dedication
MOMMY
Love of My Lifetime

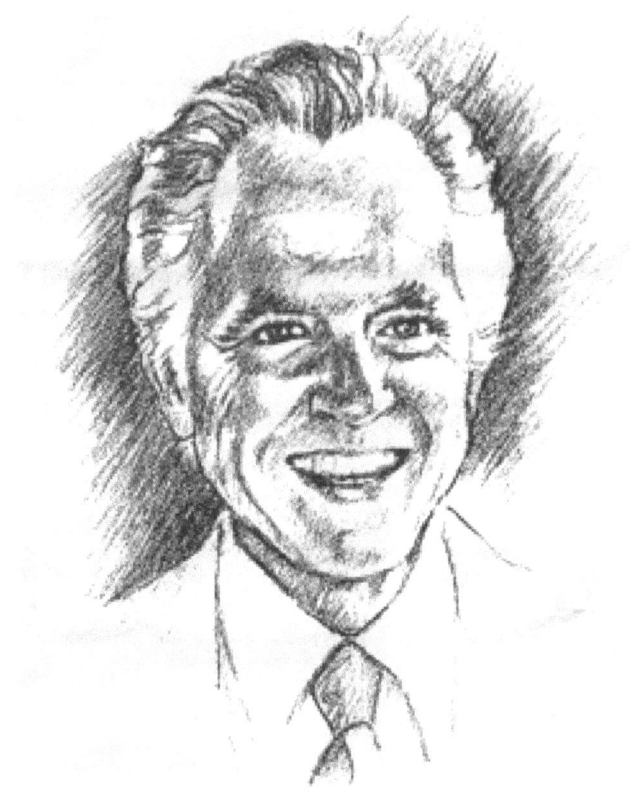

God Can Only Do For You What God Can Do Through You!

Eric Butterworth

September 12, 1916 – April 17, 2003
Minister, "Practical Mysticism"

Table of Contents

Introduction: GOD TALKS TO ME ... p.1
1. I'm Hungry! ... p.2
2. I'm Thirsty! ... p.4
3. I'm Naked! ... p.6
4. I'm Sleepy! ... p.8
5. I'm Ignorant! ... p.10
6. I'm Sick! ... p.12
7. I'm Afraid! ... p.14
8. I'm Losing Hope! ... p.16
9. I'm Lonely! ... p.18
10. I Have to Pee & Poop! ... p.20
11. I Have to Bleed for 7 Days Each Month for 33 Years! ... p.22
12. It's So Hard to Know What and How to Think! ... p.24
13. I Have Places to Go and I'm in a Hurry! ... p.26
14. I Want to Fly Like a Bird! ... p.28
15. I Want to Swim Like a Fish! ... p.30
16. I Want to Walk on the Moon! ... p.32
17. I Want to Visit the Red Planet Mars! ... p.34
18. Is There Life and a Free Lunch on Other Planets? ... p.36
19. How Do I Live a Moral Life in an Immoral Universe? ... p.38
20. I Want to Communicate with Everyone Anywhere! ... p.40
21. I Want to Shop Till I Drop! ... p.42
22. Who Am I? ... p.44
23. Who Decides Who Gets What Ideas? ... p.46
24. What is the Relationship Between Science and Religion? ... p.48
25. Did You Create the World or Did the World Create Itself? ... p.50
26. Does the Universe Have a Beginning and an End? ... p.52
27. Do You Run the World or Does the World Run Itself? ... p.54
28. When Will Nations Beat Swords into Plowshares? ... p.56
29. What About Genocide? ... p.58
30. What is the Meaning of Life? ... p.60
31. Is Life a Gift or a Punishment? ... p.62
32. Why Do We Suffer Before We Die? ... p.64
33. Is There One or Many Metaphysical Gods? ... p.66
34. What's Going on with WORLD PEACE? ... p.68
35. What is LOVE? ... p.70
36. Is My Soul Immortal? ... p.72
37. Is There Life After Death ... p.74
38. I Worked Like a DOG! ... p.76
39. Do You Hear the Voice of GOD Too? ... p.78
40. When I Pray to You, Do You Hear Me? ... p.80
41. Do You Even Exist? ... p.82
42. What Happens When You Dress Up Albert Einstein as Marilyn Monroe? ... p.84
43. What Happens When You Dress Down Albert Einstein as Marilyn Monroe? ... p.86
44. Lessons Learned? ... p.89

About the Prodigy ... pp.90–108
Gratitude ... p.108
FAN MAIL ... pp.92–103
Quotes ... pp.109, 112–113
Bookstore ... pp.110–111

"Creativity is intelligence having fun."
"Imagination is more important than knowledge. Knowledge is limited. Imagination encircles the world."
"Logic will get you from A to B. Imagination will take you everywhere."
"Creativity is seeing what others see and thinking what no one else has ever thought."
—Albert Einstein

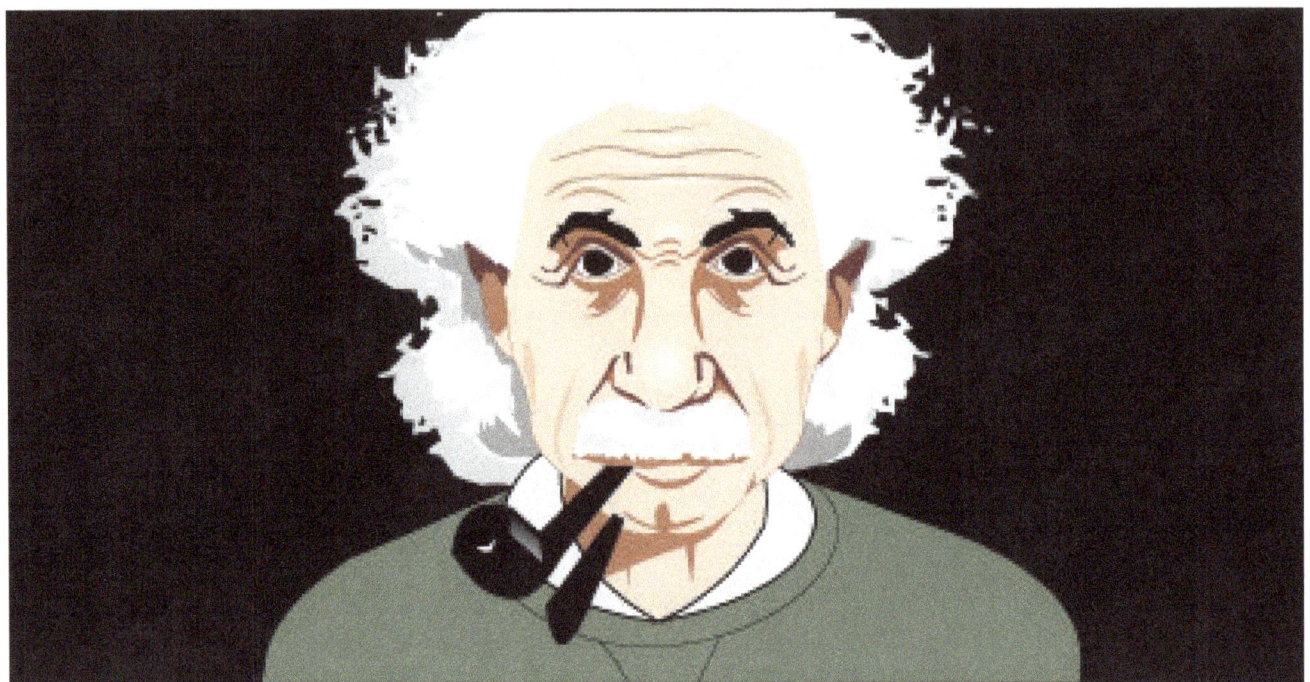

"I want to know God's thoughts— the rest are details."
—Albert Einstein
March 14, 1879 – April 18, 1955

- Jewish, German–Born Physicist
- Developed the Special and General Theories of Relativity
- Won the Nobel Prize for Physics in 1921 for His Explanation of the Photoelectric Effect

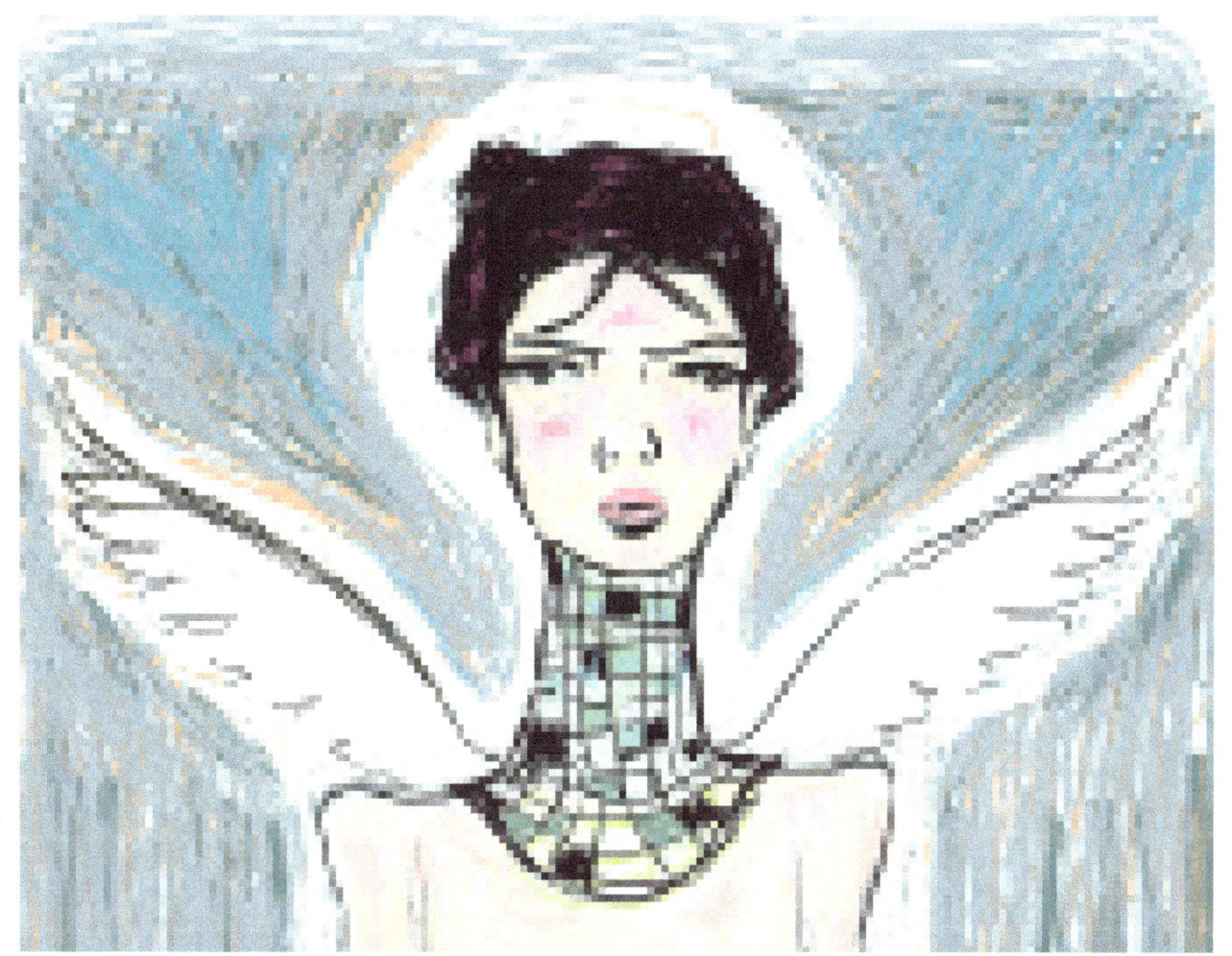

Sharon Esther Lampert

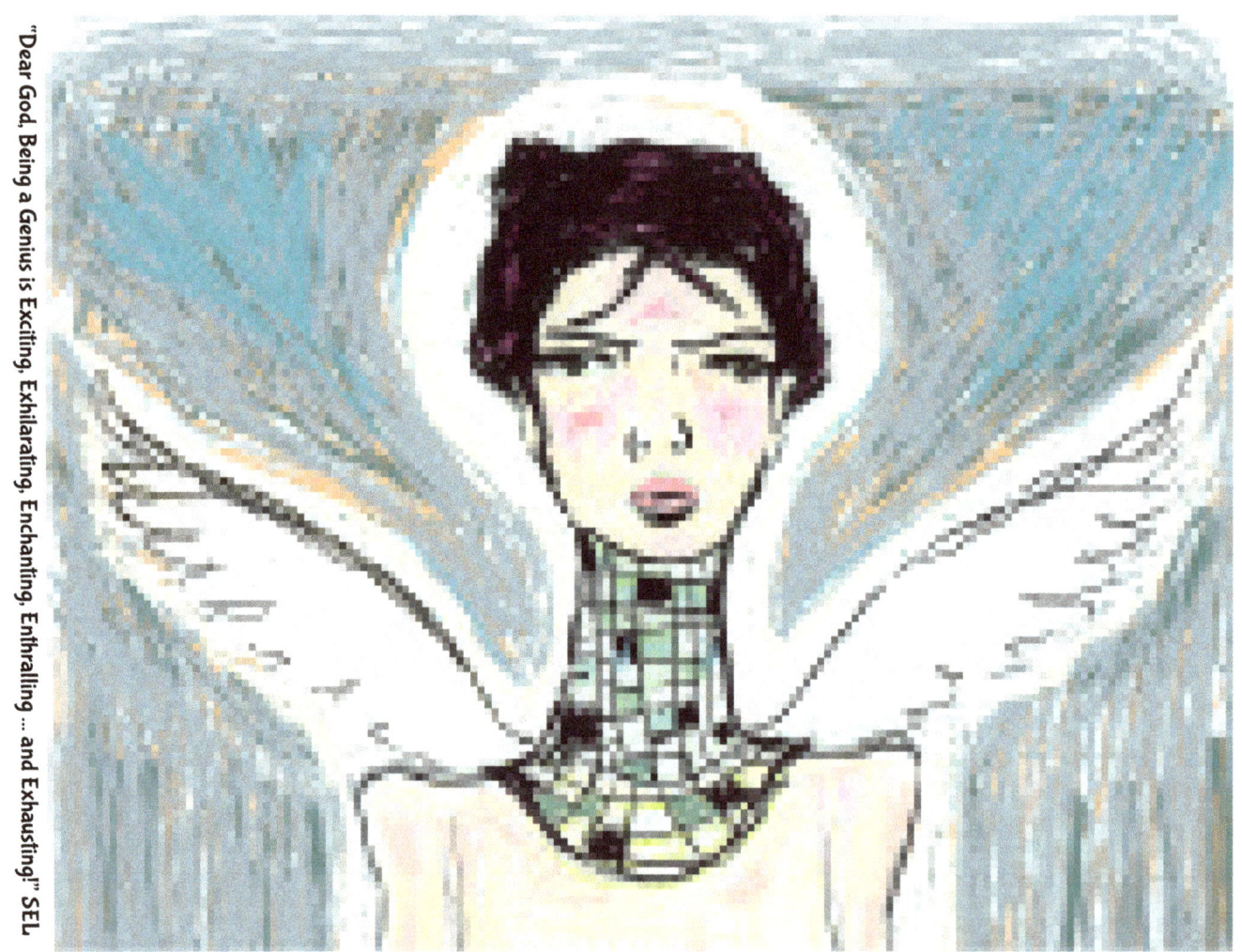

"Dear God, Being a Genius is Exciting, Exhilarating, Enchanting, Enthralling ... and Exhausting!" SEL

And God said: Dearest Sharon Esther, Do you catch my drift? You are not crazy! You are a gifted Jewish genius! Mazal Tov!

God Talks to Me: A *Working* Definition of God

Introduction

Why is it considered

NORMAL

for 7 billion people to talk to GOD in prayer; but considered

CRAZY

if GOD talks to me?

GOD talks to me every day

GOD answers every prayer! GOD answers every question!
GOD speaks a simple, but profound truth
that cannot be refuted, denied, or ignored!
Who knew GOD was such a chatterbox!

Sharon Esther Lampert
Prophet, Philosopher, Poet, Peacemaker, PHOTON & Paladin of Education, Pinup, and Prodigy
Princess Kadimah: 8TH Prophetess of Israel

1

Dear God, I'm Hungry!

God Talks to Me: A Working Definition of God

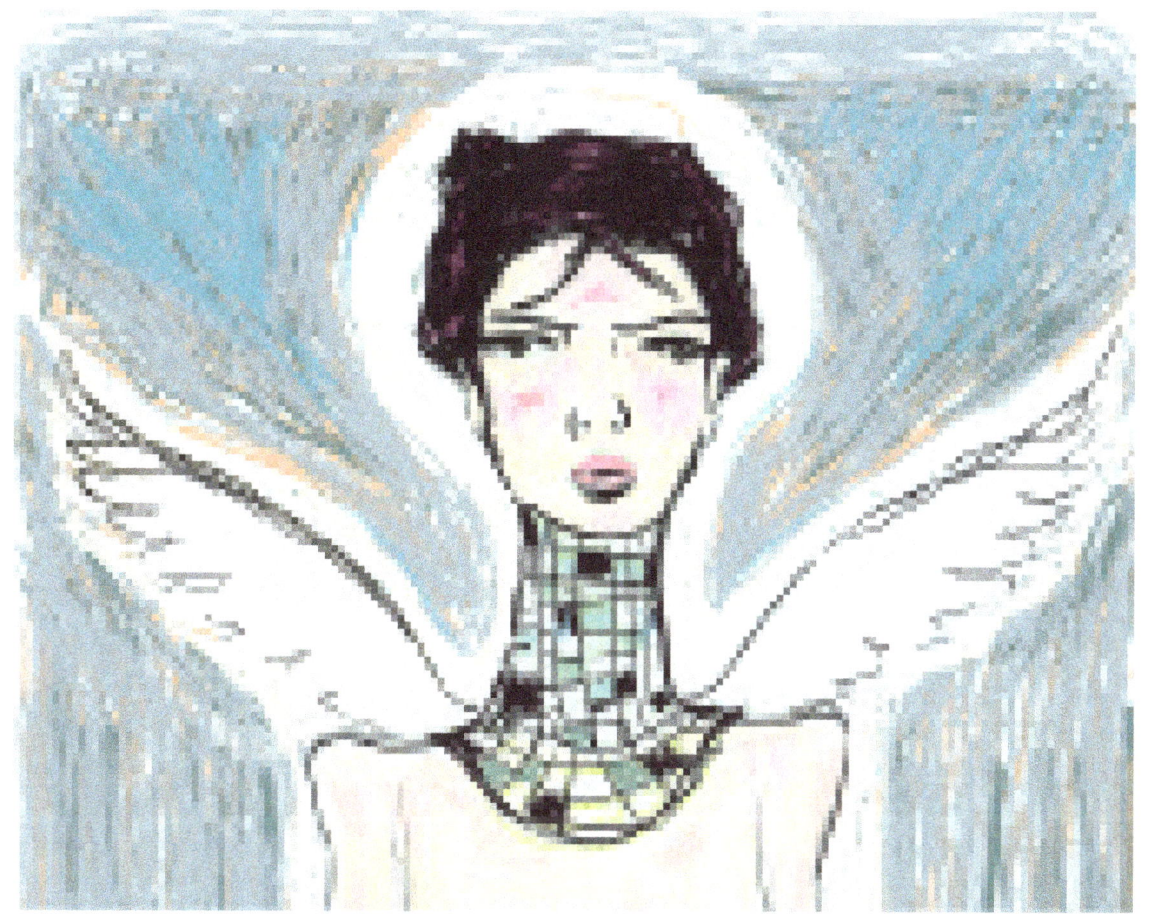

And God said:
Go to Work! Become a Farmer, Plant a Seed, and Grow an Apple Orchard!

Fiber: 4 Grams, Vitamin C: 14%, Potassium: 6%, Vitamin K: 5% Yum! Yum!

Great Works! Apple Cobbler! Apple Crisp! Apple Pie! Apple Tarte Tatin! Apple Danish!

Work a Marvel! Squeezable Peanut Butter to Feed Starving Children in Africa!

2

Dear God, I'm Thirsty!

71 Percent of Planet is Water OMG!
96.5% of Water is Salty Ocean Water OMG!

God Talks to Me: A Working Definition of God

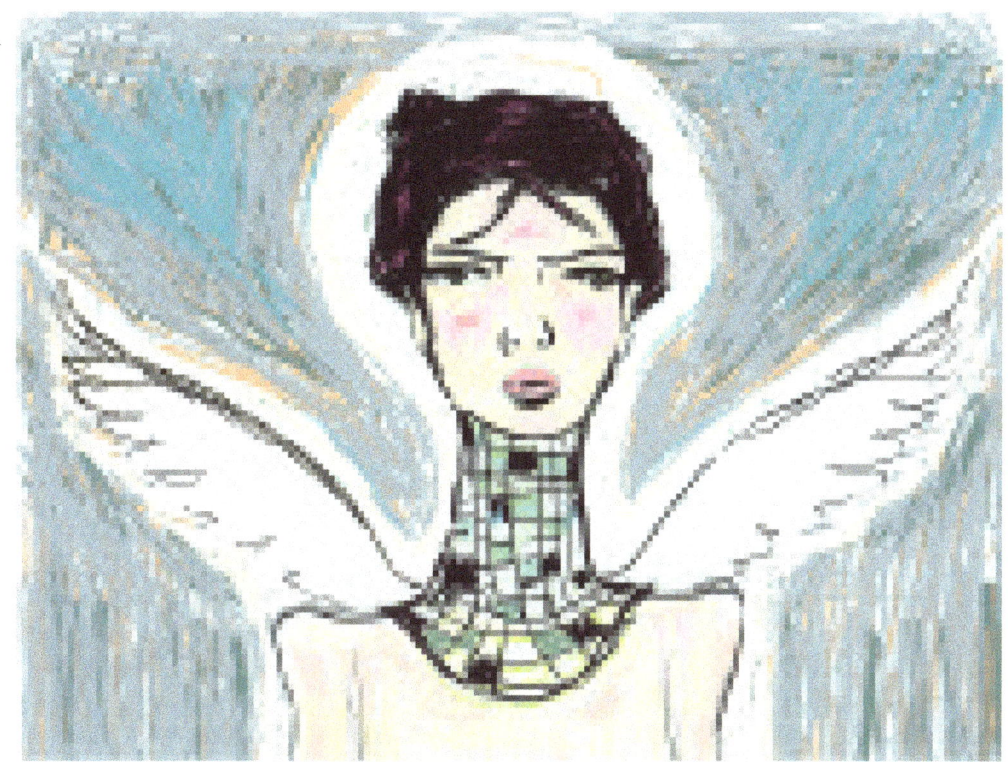

And God said:
Go to Work! 3.5% of Water is Fresh Water

30% Fresh Water is Groundwater
68% of Fresh Water is Ice and Glaciers

Great Work! Dig a Well and Filter Impurities:
Bacteria, Viruses: Fish Eggs, Baby Crabs, Plankton, Worms

Work Marvels! Satellite SMAP Soil Moisture Active Passive!

You Are Composed of 55%–70% Water, a Transport Medium for
Cells, Proteins, Glucose, Lipoproteins, and Electrolytes – Stay Hydrated!

Great Work! Bottled Water for Everyone Anywhere!

3

Dear God, I'm Naked!

God Talks to Me: A Working Definition of God

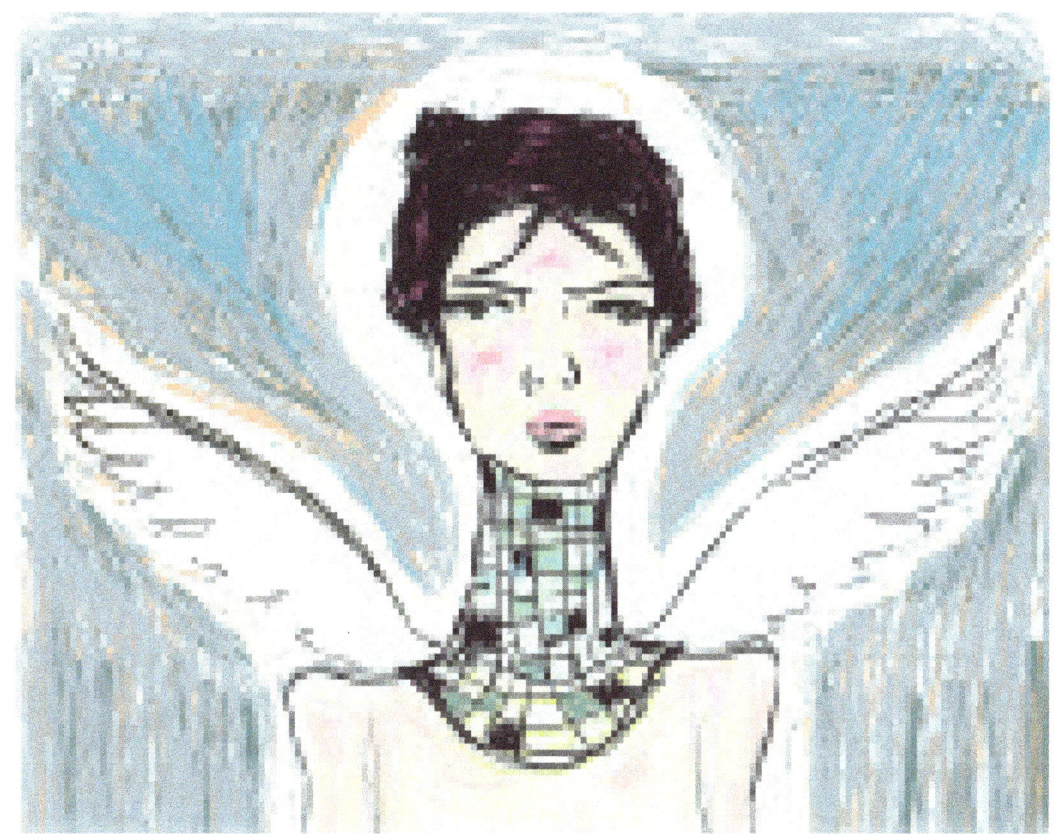

And God said:
Go to Work! Sew a Beautiful Coat, Make Spiffy Shoes, and a Matchy Purse! Wear an In-Vogue Hat with a Wide Brim!
Great Works! Casual, Classic, Costume, Fad, Formal, Haute Couture, Preppy, Trendy, and Vintage!
Work Miracles! Redesign Military & Prison Uniforms into Striped Bikinis!

4
Dear God, I'm Sleepy!
1/3 of Life Is Sleeping!

"Sleep Feels Like I'm Practicing Being Dead!"
—Philosopher Queen Sharon Esther Lampert

God Talks to Me: A Working Definition of God

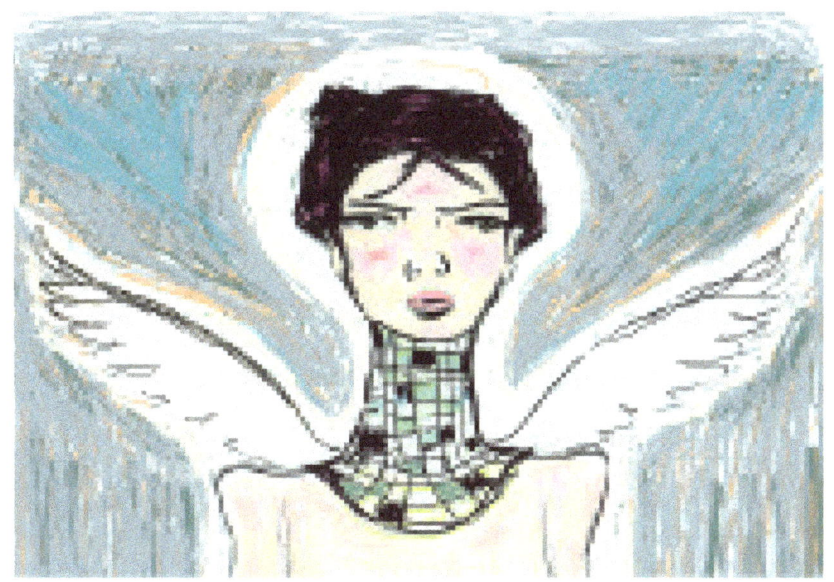

"Dear God, Why do I have to chase dustballs around a room 7 days a week? Dustballs Are Domestic Demonic Disturbances!" SEL

And God said:
Go to Work! Build a House with a Room for a Bed. Good Work! Fluffy Pillow! Work Magic Tricks! Concrete! Rubber! Plastic! Glass! Great Works! French Country, Colonial, Victorian, Tudor, Craftsman, Cottage, and Mediterranean! Work a Marvel! Electricity! Work a Mechayeh! Machines!
Refrigeration! Washer & Dryer! Dishwasher! Oven! Microwave! Toaster! Heater & Air Conditioner! Coffee Maker! Blender! Can Opener! Juicer! Lamps! Hair Dryer! Electric Toothbrush! Vacuum Cleaner! Lawnmower! Copy Machine!
Work a Miracle! Set a Regular Bedtime and Stick to It!

5

Dear God,
I'm Ignorant!
I'm Unconscious!
I'm Irrational!

I was born this way! I have to live this way! I will die this way!
It Is a 40-Year Walk in the Desert to Enlightenment!

"What Would the World Look Like if Educators Knew How to
Cultivate the Awesome Power of the Human Brain?"
—PHOTON SUPERHERO OF EDUCATION

www. SMARTGRADES BRAIN POWER REVOLUTION.com

God Talks to Me: A Working Definition of God

Read My Book!
"The Silent Crisis Destroying America's Brightest Minds"
BOOK OF THE MONTH
Alma Public Library, Wisconsin

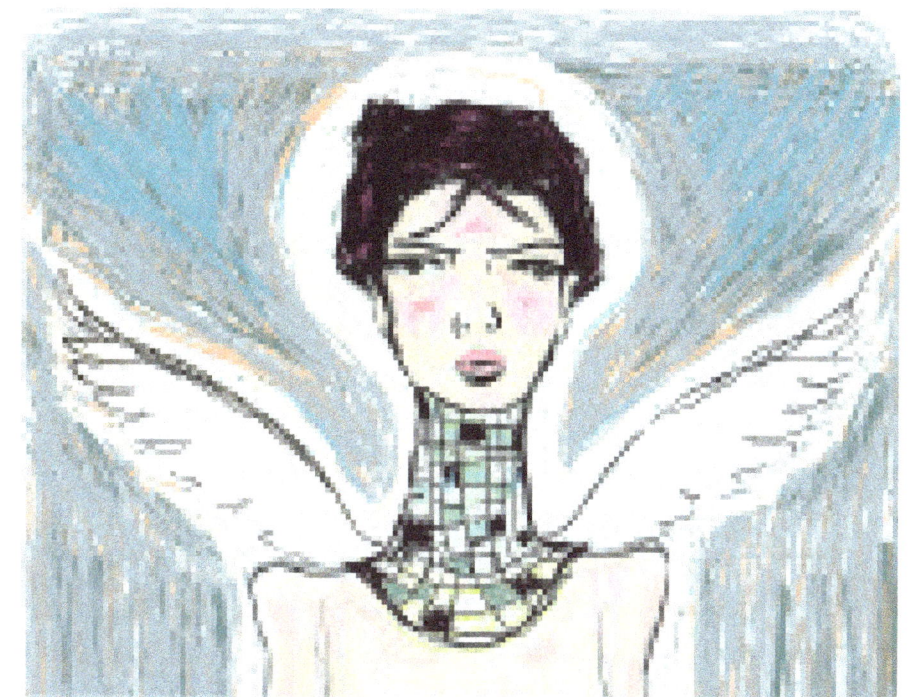

And God said:
Go to Work! Build a School, Find a Teacher, and Study Hard in School!
—Educate Mind, Body, and Soul—
Good Work! Separate Fact from Fiction!
Great Work! Transform Information into Knowledge and Knowledge into Wisdom!
Great Works! Build Libraries of FREE Books!
Work Miracles! Solve One Problem EDUCATION Save Entire World!

6

Dear God, I'm Sick!

Classic Jewish Organic Chicken Soup

In a large pot, place an organic chicken and 4 quarts of water.
Bring to a boil.
Add: onions, parsnips, celery, carrots, parsley, dill, salt, and pepper.
Partially cover the pot and simmer for 1-2 hours.
Refrigerate for 2 to 3 hours so the liquid solidifies.
When the fat rises to the top, skim it off.
Get Well Soon!

—**Philosopher Queen Sharon Esther Lampert**

God Talks to Me: A Working Definition of God

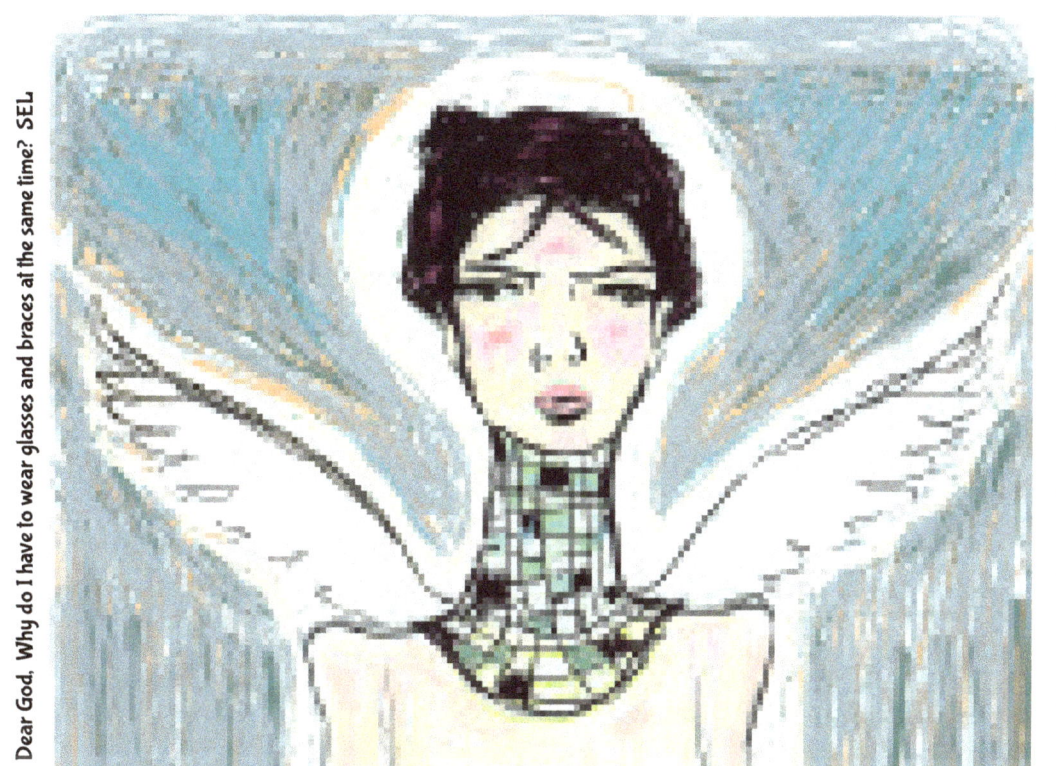

Dear God, Why do I have to wear glasses and braces at the same time? SEL

3rd Leading Cause of Death is Medical Errors! Oy Vey!

And God said:
Go to Work! Become a Doctor!
Take the Hippocratic Oath, and Build a Hospital!
Take X–RAYS! Develop Vaccines! Brew Medicines!
Great Works: Antibiotics, Microscopes, Thermometers, Stethoscopes!
Work Magic Tricks! Stem Cells, Regeneration, and Rebirth!
Work Marvels! Immunotherapy – Cancer Free!
Work a Miracle! Do No Harm! Help the Body Heal Itself!

7

Dear God, I'm Afraid!

(Worried, Anxious, Stressed, Depressed, and PSTD)

"When you know the notes to sing, you can sing most anything!"
— Julie Andrews, "Sound of Music" – Oscar Hammerstein

God Talks to Me: A Working Definition of God

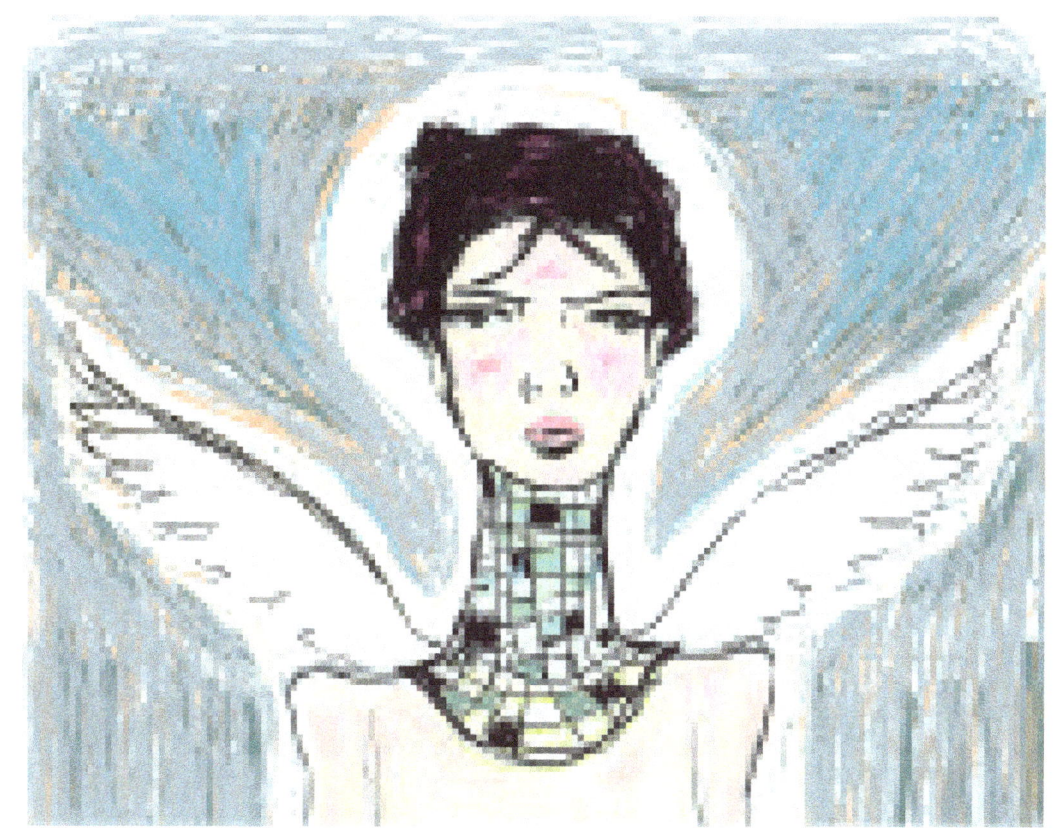

And God said:
Go to Work! Write a Violin Concerto!
Listen to Felix Mendelssohn, E Minor, Op.64, Allegro Molto Appassionato

Great Work! The Chromatic Scale of 12 Notes!
Work Magic! Strings! Brass! Woodwinds! Percussion!
Marvelous Works! Pop! Rock! Classical! Jazz! Blues! Country! Broadway!
Work a Miracle! Listen to Your (My) Inner Voice: Do! Re! Mi! Fa! So! La! Ti!

8
Dear God, I'm Losing Hope!

"Meditation, Mindfulness, Mantra, and Music Mitigates MADNESS!"
—Philosopher Queen Sharon Esther Lampert

God Talks to Me: A Working Definition of God

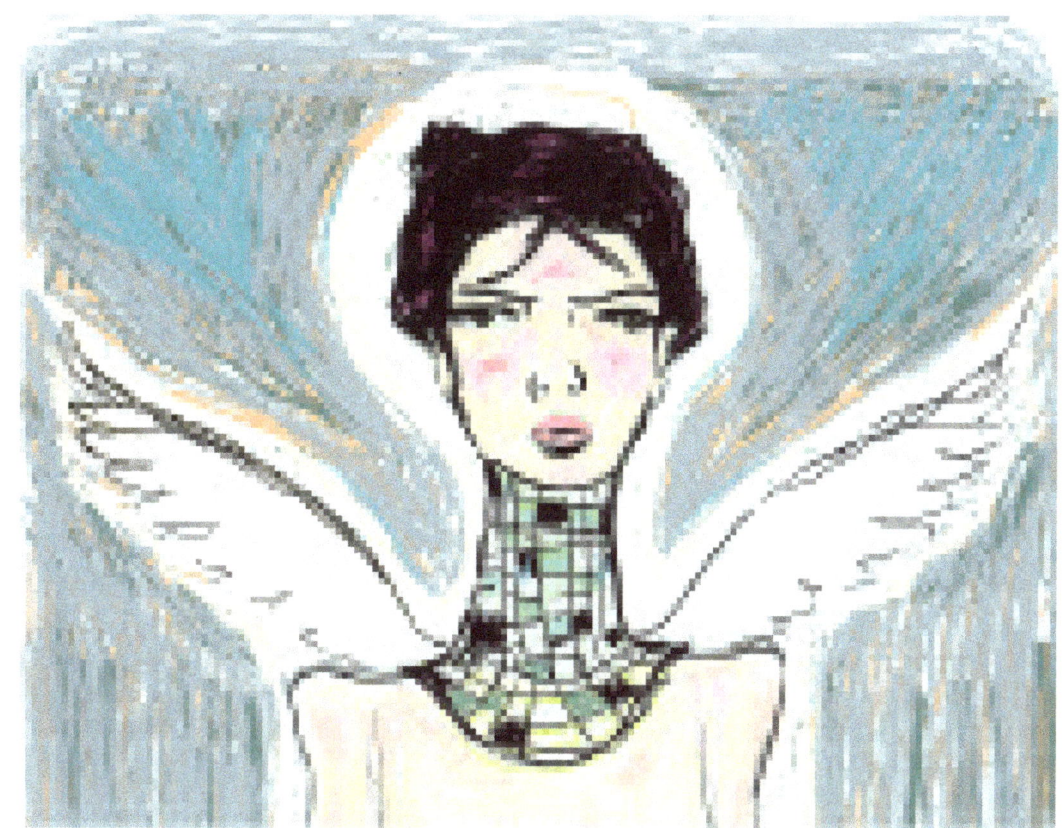

And God said:
Go to Work! Count Your Blessings!
Practice Gratitude! Practice Meditation!
Create a Mantra: "Find the Light & Live in the Light!"
Practice Mindfulness: BE HERE NOW!

9

Dear God, I'm Lonely!

8 Billion Workers! (2022)
Asia: 4.5 Billion Workers! (China: 1.4 Billion Workers!, India (1.4 Billion Workers!)
Africa: 1.4 Billion Workers!
Americas: 1 Billion Workers!
Europe: 750 Million Workers!

1804: **1 Billion Workers!**
1927: 2 Billion (123 years later))
1960: 3 Billion (33 years later)
1974: 4 Billion (14 years later)
1987: 5 Billion (13 years later)
1999: 6 Billion (12 years later)
2011: 7 Billion (12 years later)
2023: 8 Billion (12 years later)

"Loneliness Is Death! Solitude Is Divine!"
—Philosopher Queen Sharon Esther Lampert

God Talks to Me: A Working Definition of God

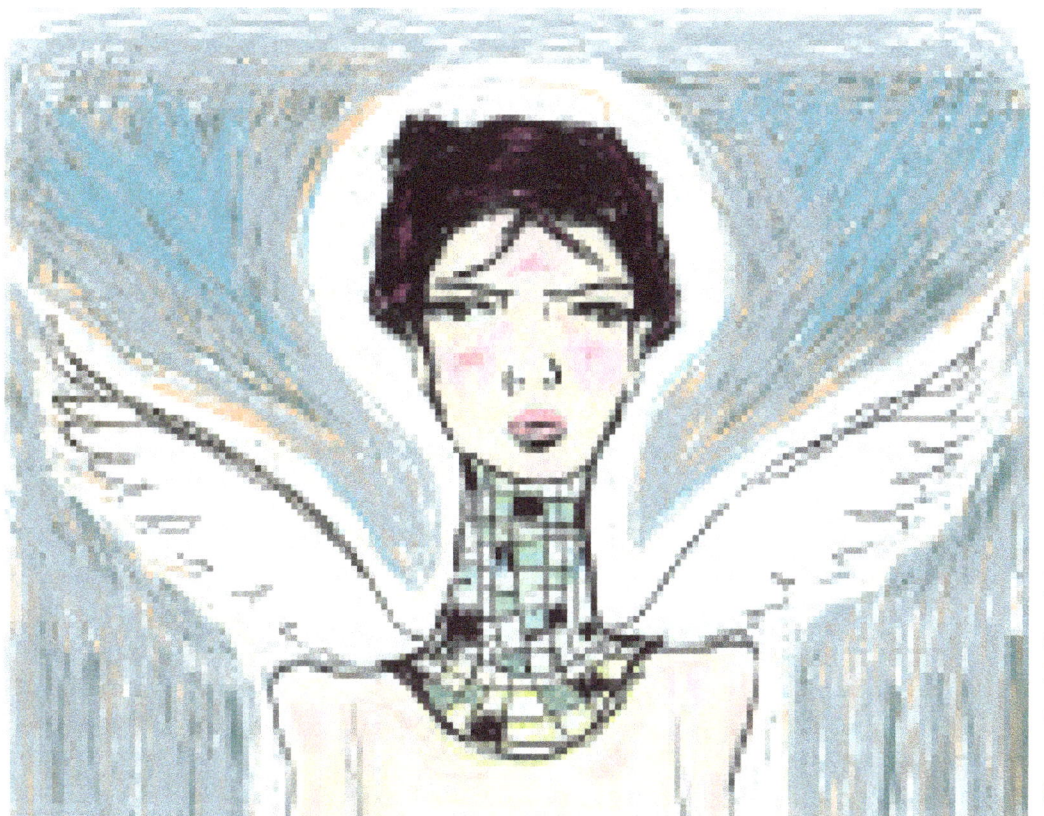

MEWOW!
Read Children's Book: "SCHMALTZY: In America, Even a Cat Can Have a Dream!"

Philosopher Queen Sharon Esther Lampert

"Dear God, Why did my cat have to die?" (4th grade) SEL

And God said:
Go to Work! Share the Heavy Workload!
Build a Family: Mate, Kids, and Loyal Pets!

Good Work! Dog Fetches Newspaper, Remote Control, and Frisbee!
Great Works! Therapy Dogs! Service Dogs! Search & Rescue Dogs!
Herding Dogs! Military Dogs! Police Dogs!
Work Marvels! SCHMALTZY: World Famous Piano-Playing Cat!

10

Dear God, I have to pee & poop 3X day!

Poop per day is 15 ounces (2 poops per day)
Poop per week per person is 6 pounds
Poop per year per person is 320 pounds

"I recommend Angel Soft's "Fresh Lavender" Toilet Paper!"
—Philosopher Queen Sharon Esther Lampert

God Talks to Me: A Working Definition of God

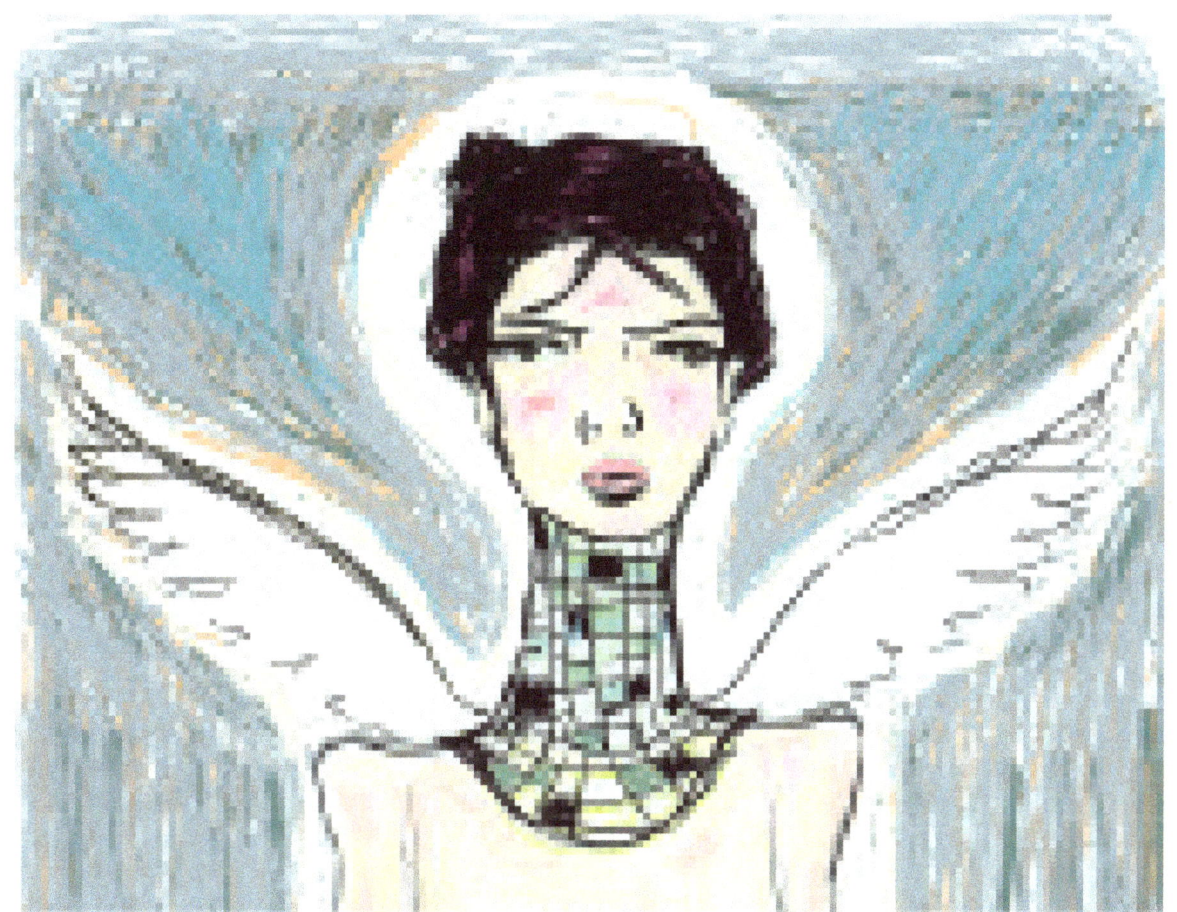

And God said:
Go to Work! Make a Toilet, a Treatment Plant, and Toilet Paper: Soft, Extrasoft, and Scented!

Great Work! Indoor Plumbing!

Work a Miracle! In 60 Months, 100 Million Toilets are Built for 600 Million People in India! (2019).

11

Dear God, I have to bleed 5–7 days each month for 33 years!

Woe is Me! Painful Childbirth!
Woe is Me! Wife & Woman's Work!
Woe is Me! Working Woman & Half the Pay!
Woe is Me! 10 Years & 34 Symptoms of Menopause!
Woe is Me! 100 Million Girls Cannot Go to School (Malala.org)!
Woe is Me! Reproductive Freedom: Incest, Rape, Birth Defects & Teenage Pregnancy!
Woe is METOO! 14 Global Catastrophes of Violence Against Women!
—Philosopher Queen Sharon Esther Lampert

God Talks to Me: A Working Definition of God

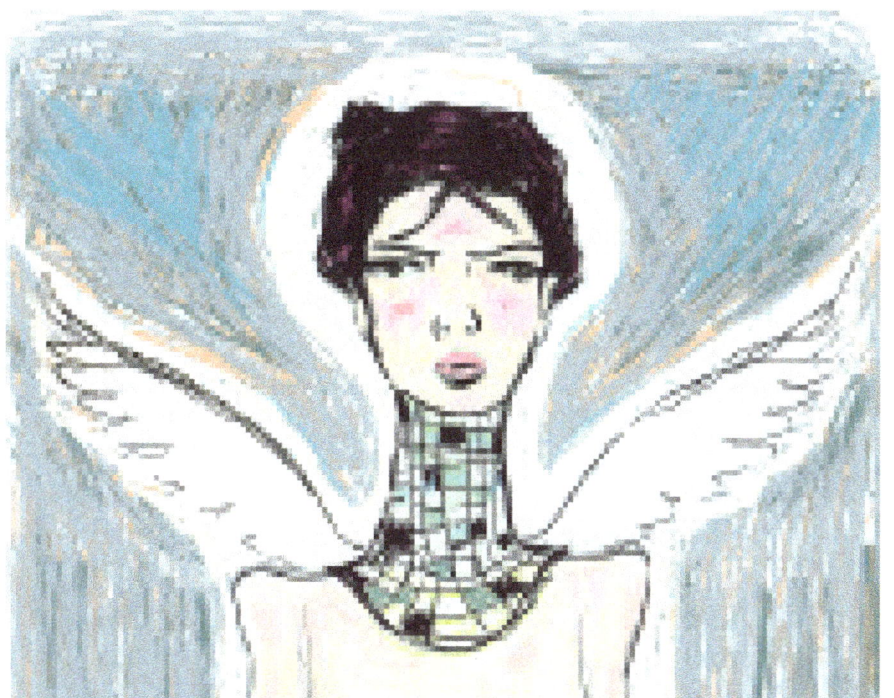

Read My Books:

"Silly Little Boys: 40 Rules of Manhood!"

"Women Have All the Power — But Have Never Learned How to Use It"

Philosopher Queen
Sharon Esther Lampert

"Dear God, Please don't give me GIANT BREASTS like Mommy and Grandma!" (4th Grade) SEL

And God said: Go to Work! Make a Tampon and a Napkin. Use both!

Women Have All The Power — But Have Never Learned How to Use It!
You Are Not a Sideshow — You Are the Main Attraction!
Your Vagina Is the Gatekeeper, the Portal for All Humanity!
Magnificent Work! Cliteracy!
The Only Organ in the Human Body Whose Sole Purpose
Is Female Sexual Orgasmic Pleasure! Fantasy at Work! Vibrators!

12

Dear God, It's so hard to know how to think, and what to think!

"Imperfect World, Imperfect Problem, Imperfect Solution"
—Philosopher Queen Sharon Esther Lampert

God Talks to Me: A Working Definition of God

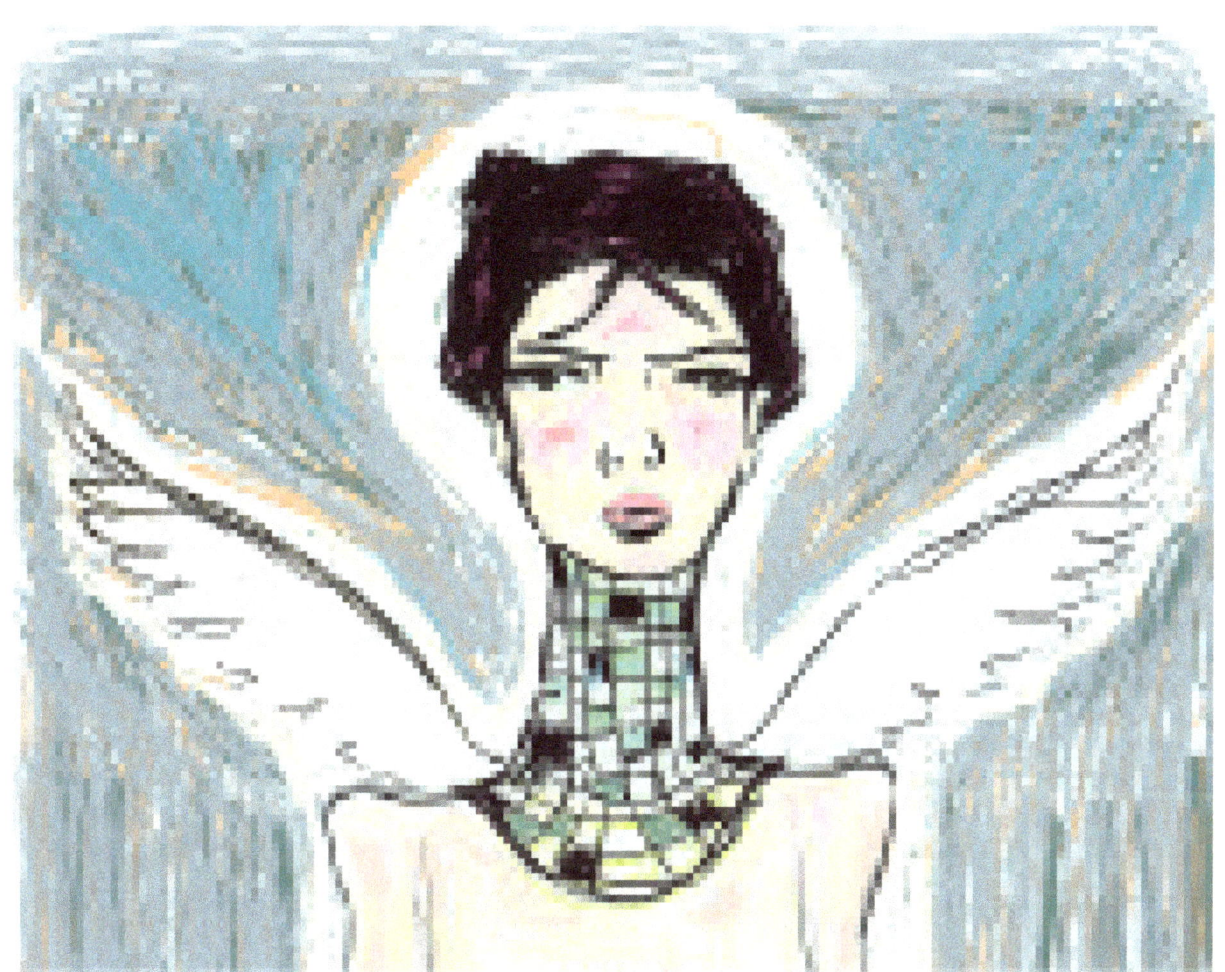

And God said: Go to Work!
There is One Global Enemy: IGNORANCE
The Learning Curve is Steep: GOOGLE 50X a DAY!
"Global Organization of Oriented Group Language of Earth"

13

Dear God,
I have places to go, people to see, and I'm in a hurry!

God Talks to Me: A Working Definition of God

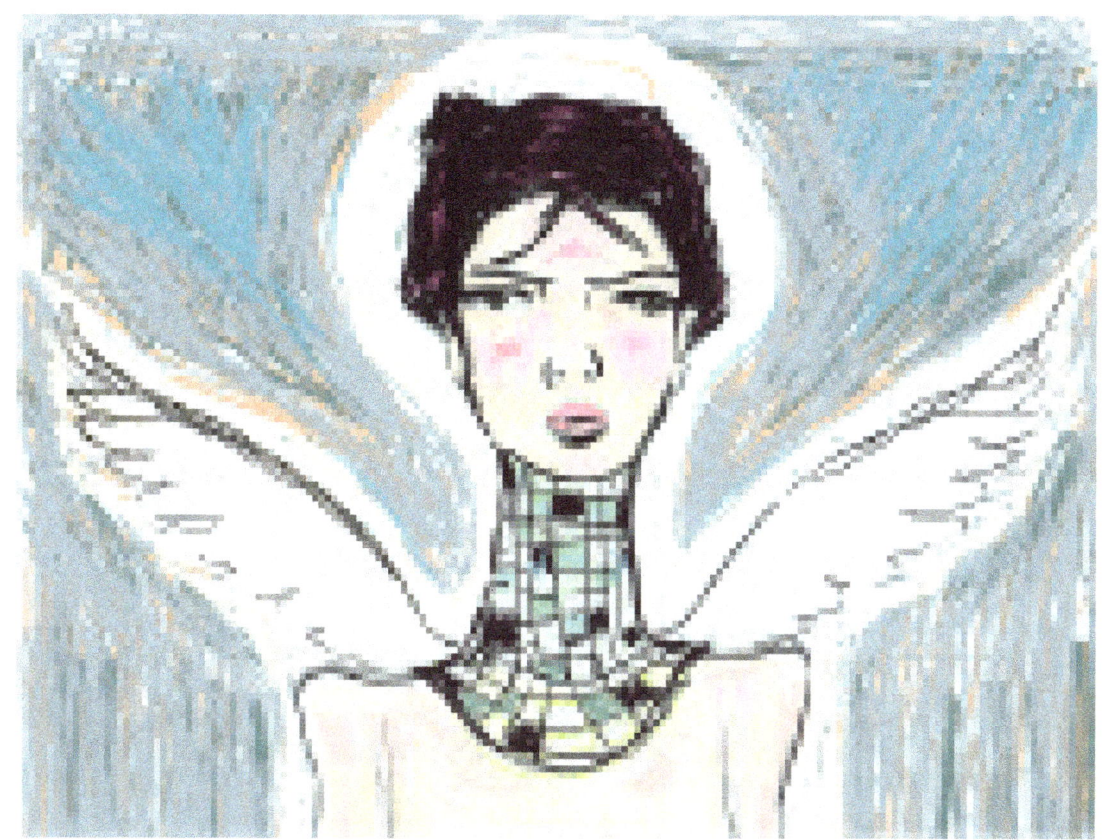

And God said: Go to Work! Stop Horsing Around!

Build a Car, Bus, and Train Above Ground, and Build a Subway Below Ground! Good Work! Elevators! Great Works! Build Beautiful Bustling Bridges: Beam, Truss, Cantilever, Arch, Suspension, and Cable! Work Marvels! Fossil Fuels: Oil, Coal, and Natural Gas!

14

Dear God, I want to fly like a bird!

God Talks to Me: A Working Definition of God

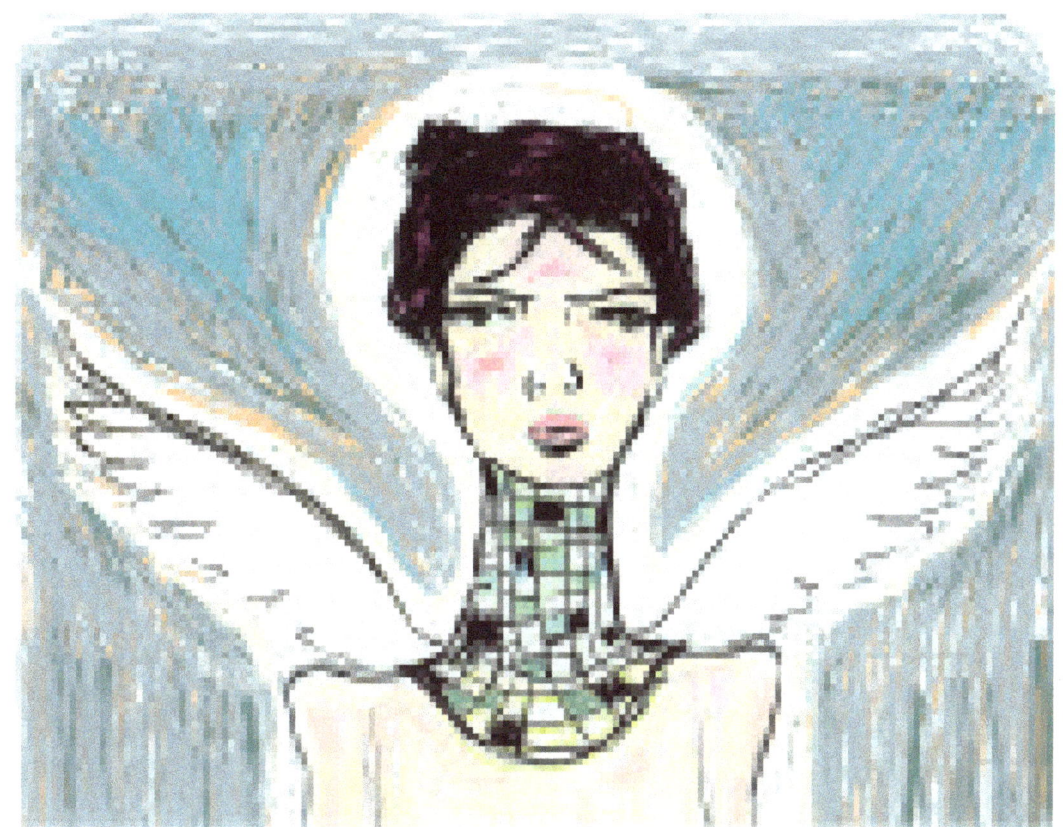

And God said:
Go to Work! Become a Pilot!
Build an Airplane, Helicopter, Glider, and Kite to Soar High into the Sky of Cumulus, Stratus, and Cirrus Clouds!
Great Work! Renewable Clean Energy Combats Climate Crisis!
Work Marvels! ORCA Captures 4000 Metric Tons of CO_2/year!
Work Miracles! Come Visit Me in Your Head, Heart, and Heaven!

15

Dear God, I want to swim like a fish!

God Talks to Me: A Working Definition of God

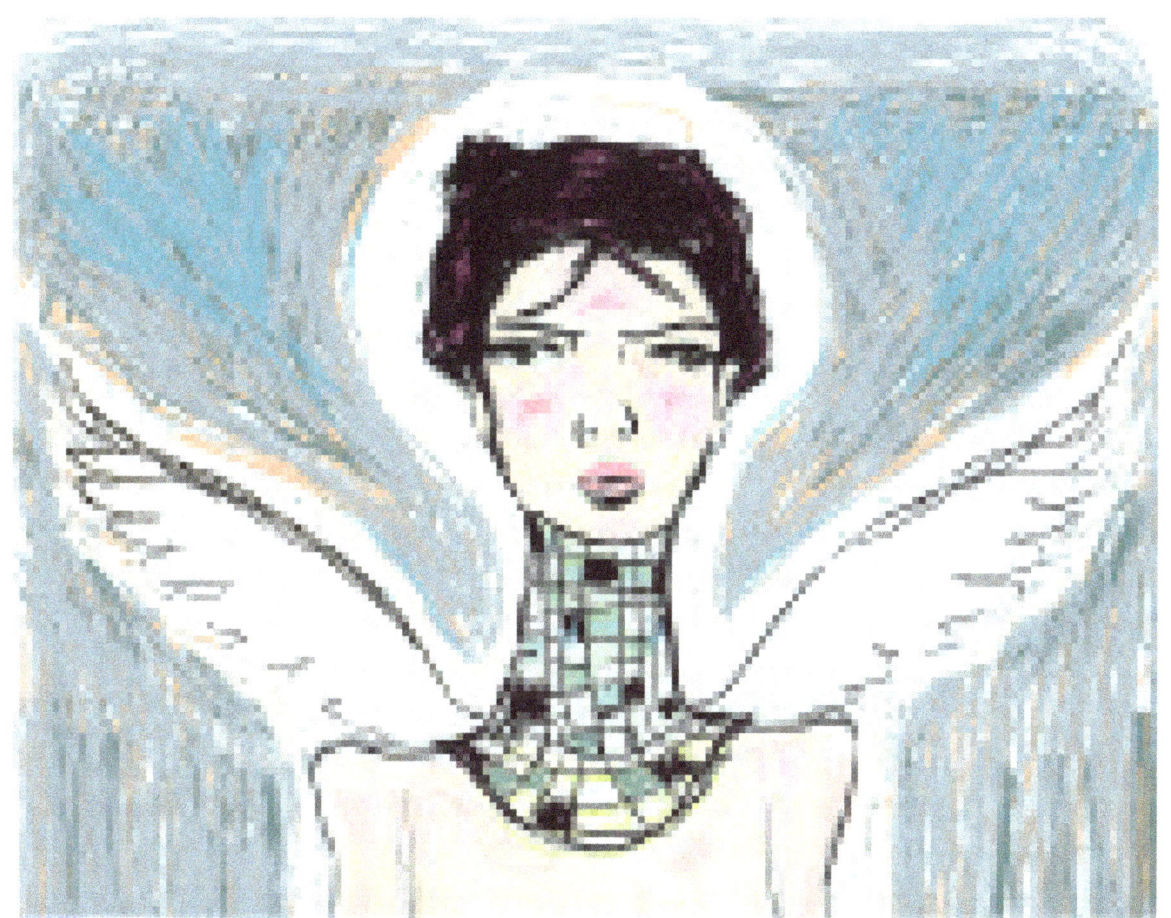

And God said:
Go to Work! Become a Scuba Diver! Build a Raft, Boat, Ship and Submarine to Sail Above and Below the Azure Seas!
Work a Miracle! Protect My Oceans from Plastic Pollution!

16

Dear God, I want to walk on the moon!

God Talks to Me: A Working Definition of God

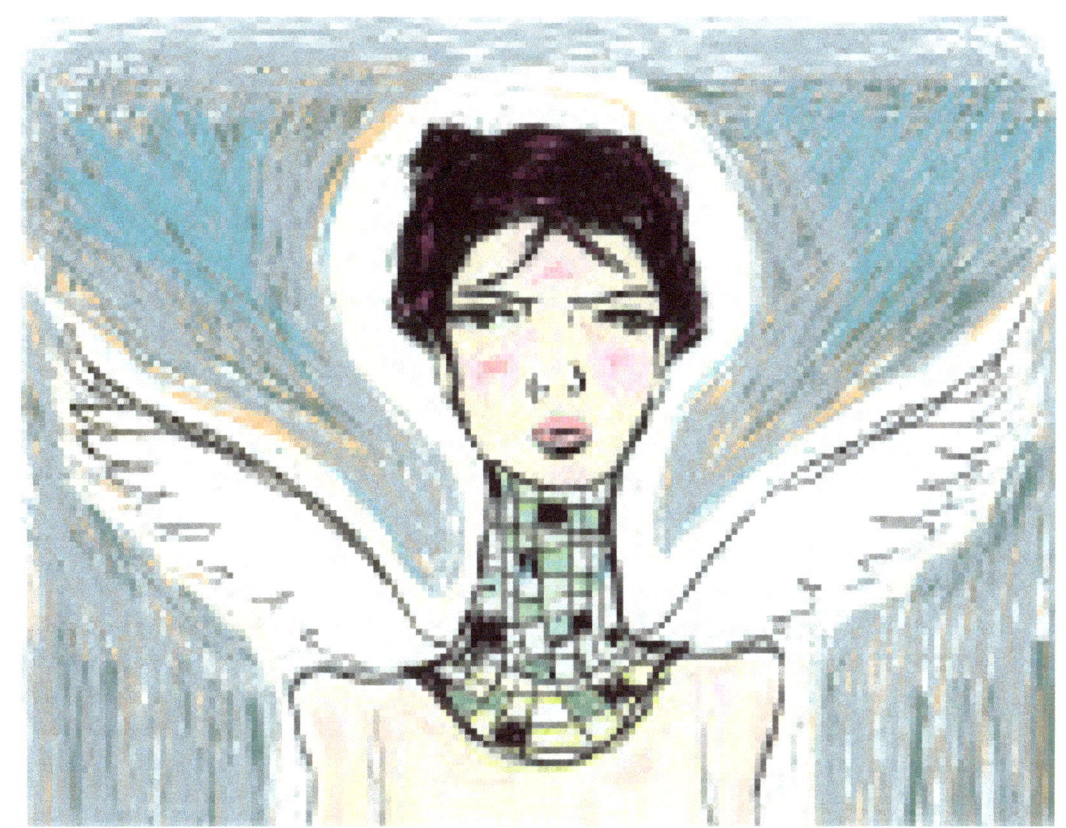

And God said: Become an Astronaut! Go to Work! Build a Rocket Ship and Lift Off!

USA, July 20, 1969 — Apollo 11: Neil Armstrong & Buzz Aldrin

Apollo 12 — Apollo 17: 12 USA Astronauts Landed on Moon!

Conrad; Bean; Shepard Jr.; Mitchell; Scott; Irwin; Young; Duke; Cernan; Schmitt

GODSPEED! GO! DO! ARTEMIS 2028!

17

Dear God, I want to visit the red planet Mars!

"7 months before, the US predicted a Mars landing on February 18th, 2021 OMG!"

—Philosopher Queen Sharon Esther Lampert

God Talks to Me: A Working Definition of God

35

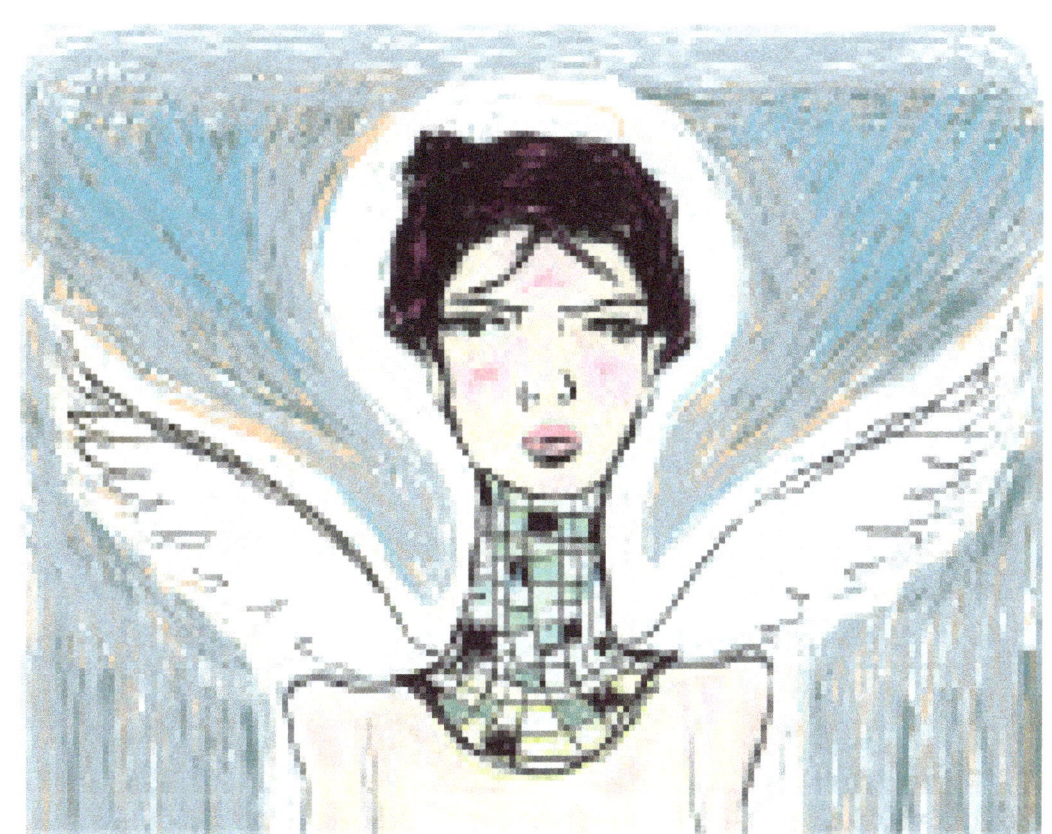

And God said: Go to Work! Orbiters, Landers, Rovers

Nine Landings! Viking 1 & Viking 2 (1976), Pathfinder (1997), Spirit and Opportunity (2004), Phoenix (2008), Curiosity (2012), InSight (2018), and Rover Perseverance (Feb 18, 2021)!

18

Dear God, Is There Life and a Free Lunch on Other Planets?

God Talks to Me: A Working Definition of God

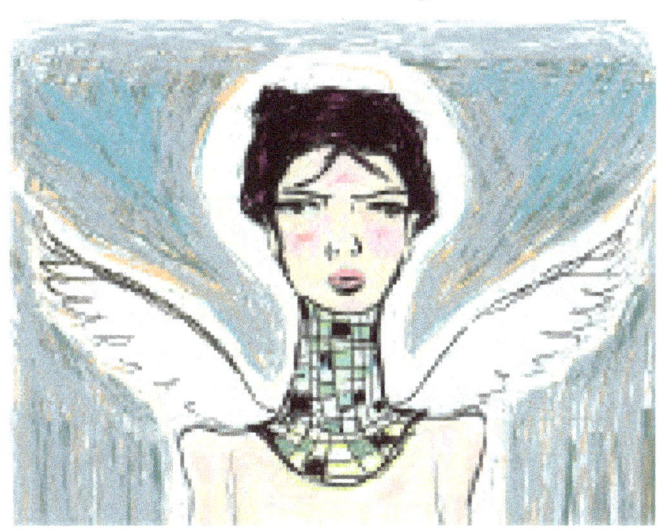

And God said: Go to Work!
Find a Planet with Life and a Free Lunch!
There Are 8.7 Million Life Forms on Planet Earth, and Most Fear, Hate, and Eat the Other to Survive!
Good Work! Earth Revolves Around Sun!
Great Work! Solar System of 9 Planets!
Venus, Jupiter, Mercury, Saturn, Earth, Mars, Uranus, Neptune, and Pluto
Work Marvels! 7 Galaxies!
Andromedia, Canis, Cygnus, Maffei, Magellanic, Milky Way, and Virgo
Marvelous Work! The International Space Station of 16 Countries!
Magnificent Work! DART: Double Asteroid Redirection Test!
For a Rogue Asteroid Hurtling Toward Earth! Oy Vey!
Work a Miracle! James Webb Space Telescope!

19

Dear God, How Do I Live a Moral Life in an Immoral Universe?

OMG! You Can Eat Your Own Children for Lunch!

"You can do it all right — and get it all wrong!
You can do it all wrong — and get it all right!"
—Philosopher Queen Sharon Esther Lampert

God Talks to Me: A Working Definition of God

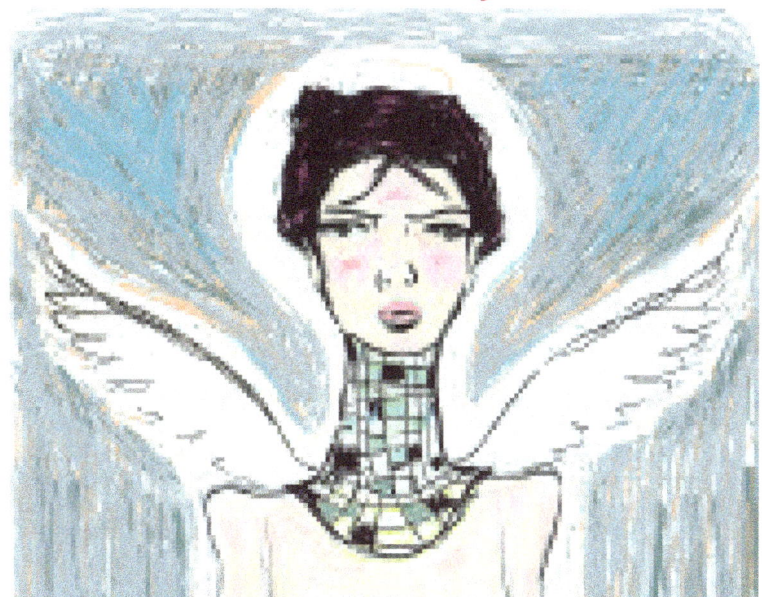

MALALA MESSIAH
(Jesus Christ!)

* Persecution
* Crucifixion
* Resurrection
* Redemption
* Phoenix Rising!
* Messiah

And God said:
Go to Work! Roll the Dice!
8 Probabilities!

1. Good Goes to Good
2. Good Goes to Bad
3. Good Goes to Good & Bad
4. Good Goes to Nothing
5. Bad Goes to Bad
6. Bad Goes to Good
7. Bad Goes to Good and Bad
8. Bad Goes to Nothing

Meaningful Work!
(1) Good Goes to Evil   (2) Evil Goes to Good and Great   (3) Good Goes to Great!

(1) Malala Went to School and Was Shot in the Head by the Taliban.
(2) After 12+ Painful Surgeries, Malala Earns a First-Rate UK Education and a Nobel Prize!
(3) Malala's Life Is Dedicated to Helping 100 Million Girls Learn. A Mighty Worker!

#IAMMALALA   #LETGIRLSLEARN   #SMARTGRADESBRAINPOWER

20

Dear God, I want to communicate with everyone anywhere!

God Talks to Me: A Working Definition of God

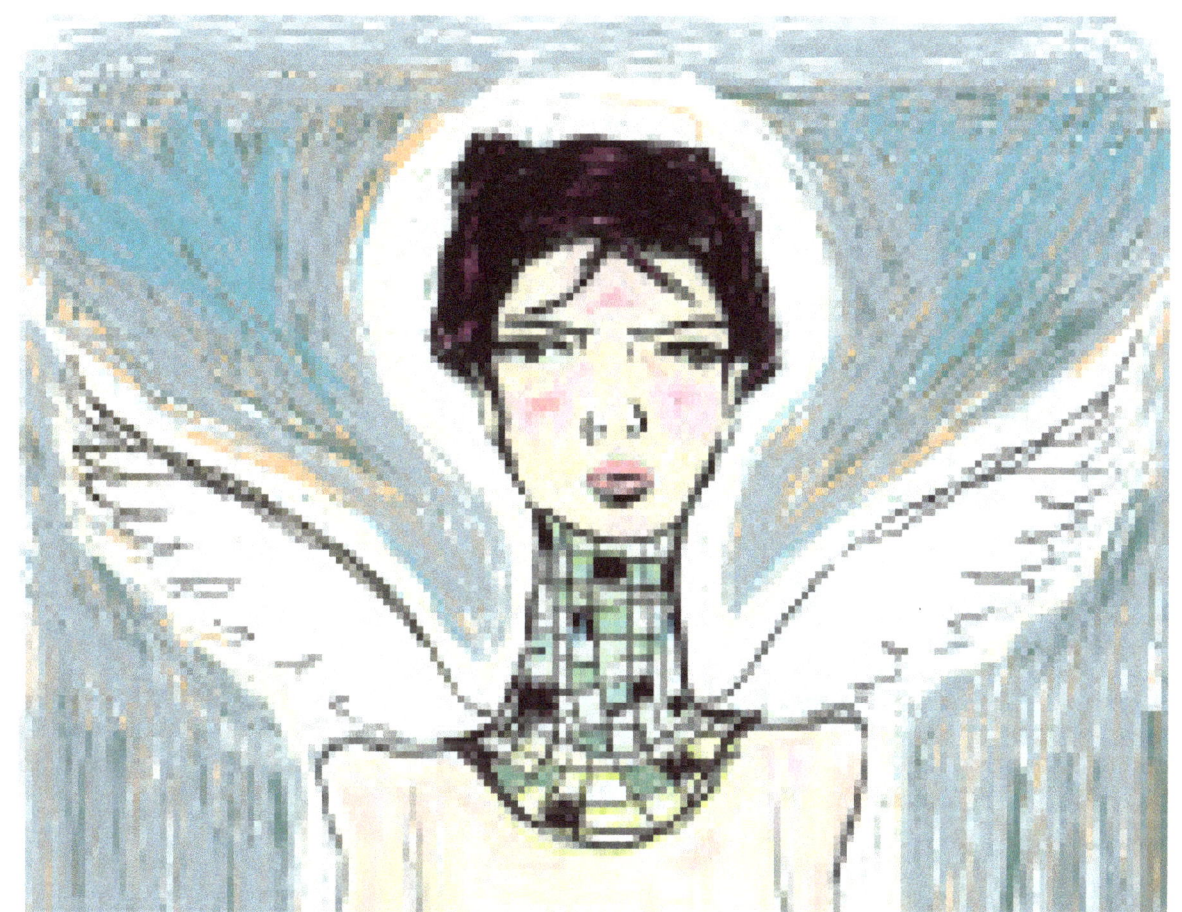

And God said:
Go to Work! Build an APPLE Computer with ADOBE Software!
Build an Internet and Send an E-Mail to Everyone Anywhere!
Do Not Forget to Back Up Your Work!
Marvelous Works! Semiconductors! AI!

21

Dear God, I Want to Shop Till I Drop!

God Talks to Me: A *Working* Definition of God

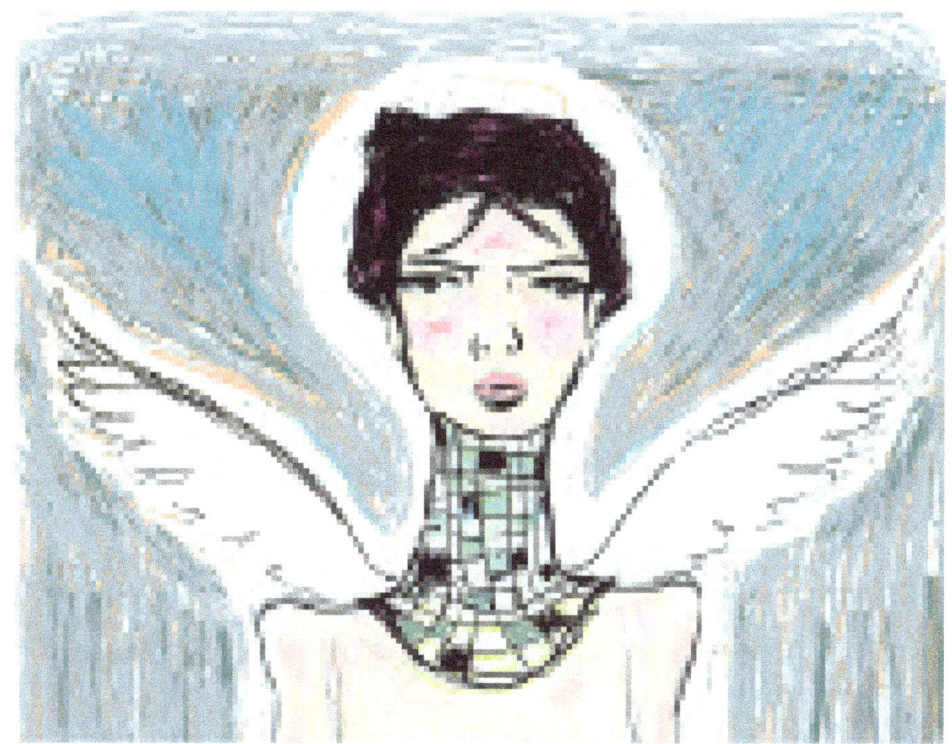

And God said: Go to Work! AMAZON

On a Global Scale, Order Everything from Anywhere with the Click of a Computer Mouse — and Have All of It Delivered to Your Front Door! If You Ordered the Wrong Size — Return All of It with Another Click of the Computer Mouse!
Work a Mechaiah! The Best for Less!
Work Miracles! 2–Day Prime and Free Shipping!

22

Dear God, Who Am I?

Fertilized Egg to Zygote (Cells Divide) to Embryo (Cells Differentiate) to Fetus to Me!

"The two most important days in your life are the day you are born and the day you find out why."
– Mark Twain

God Talks to Me: A Working Definition of God

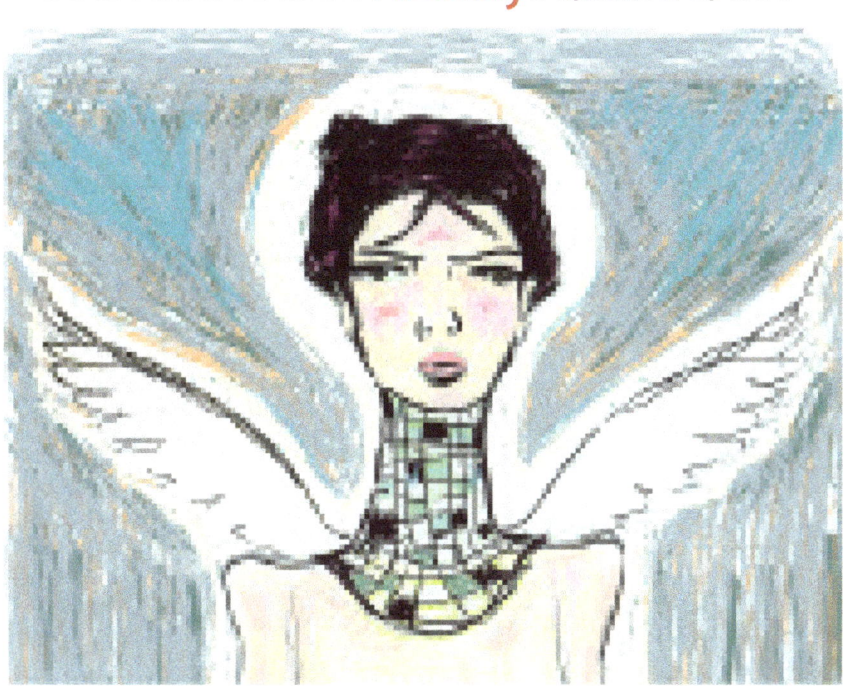

Read My Book:

SPERM MANIFESTO
10 Rules for the Road

Philosopher Queen
Sharon Esther Lampert

Read My Book:
DESTINY
— Written in Letter D

Desire
Dreams
Decisions
Directions
Determination
Deadlines
DESTINY

Philosopher Queen
Sharon Esther Lampert

The Awesome Art of Alliteration Using One Letter of the Alphabet

And God said:
Go to Work! Break Out of Your Birth Bubble!
We Live Life by Default — Later by Design!

You Play the Cards You Are Dealt — What You Do
with the Cards You Are Dealt Determines Your Destiny!
Great Work! Upward Climb Against Gravity in Uterus!
Great Work! 9 Month Incubation in Womb!
Work Marvels! MY DAY! MY DREAM! MY DESTINY!
Work a Miracle! DARE TO DREAM!
Work Magic! LIVE YOUR TRUTH!

23

Dear God,
Who decides who gets what ideas?

My metaphysical mind is full of brilliant ideas!

Age 9:
Dear Sharon Esther,
THE QUEEN HAS ARRIVED!
My Daughter is a Poet, Philosopher, and Teacher.
Sharon is the Princess & the Pea.
BEAUTY & BRAINS!
XOXO
—MOMMY

God Talks to Me: A Working Definition of God

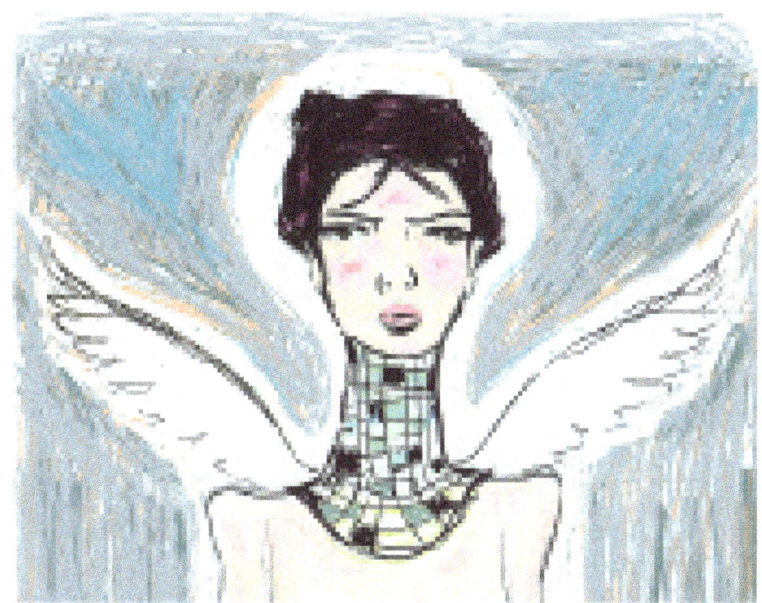

And God said: PRODIGY
Go to Work! Measure Twice and Cut Once!
The Fine Line Between Genius and Insanity Is Organization!
— Make a Plan in Place on Paper —
Go to Work! Writing Is Rewriting! Pencils, Pens, and Paper!
Great Works! 7000 Spoken Languages and 7000 Translators!
Work Miracles! Numbers, Numerals, and Calculators!
Do the Math: Algebra, Geometry, and Calculus!
Make Time Work for You!
Use My Time Shifts: 5–9 a.m., 9–12 p.m., 12–3 p.m., 3–6 p.m., 6–9 p.m.
Beautiful Works! Cuckoo Clocks, Hourglass, Sundial, Alarm Clocks, Timers, Stop Watches, Wristwatches, and APPLE Watch!

24

Dear God,

What Is the Relationship Between Science & Religion? Between Physical World & Metaphysical World?

Q. Why do you wake up Sharon Esther in the middle of the night to write the whole book?

Read My Children's Book:
"Why Isn't Sharon Sleeping?"

God Talks to Me: A Working Definition of God

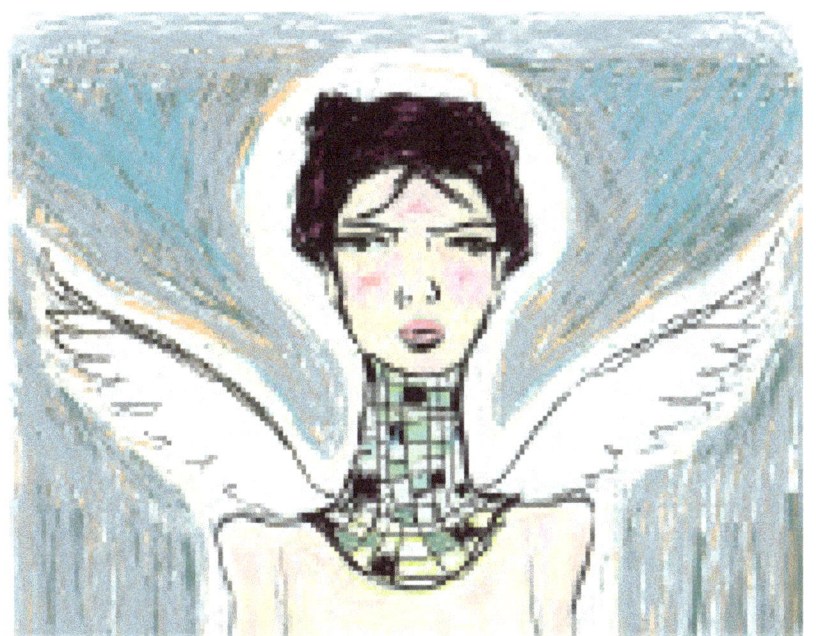

There are 2 Universes: Physical and Metaphysical They Are Inextricably Linked

Ideas, Imagination Intuition, and Insight Exist in My Metaphysical Universe

The physical world provides the raw materials. The metaphysical world transforms the raw materials: mind, ideas, thoughts

Aristotelian Syllogism

And God said:
You Think Therefore I Am and God Is!
There Is a Physical and Metaphysical Universe!
Go to Work! Religion Is Faith and Science Is Facts
Go to Work! Faith and Facts Always Work in Unison
Go to Work! Science & Religion Always Work in Unison
Your Mind (Unconscious and Conscious), Your Thoughts, and Ideas Are Invisible and Intangible Entities Beyond Scientific Inquiry that Exist in the Metaphysical Universe.
Religion has Dominion Over the Metaphysical Universe.
Science has Dominion Over the Physical Universe.
Work a Miracle! Learn to Show Each Other Respect!
It takes FACTS to build an airplane —but FAITH to take a ride across the sky!

25

Dear God,
Did you create the world or did the world create itself?

Dark Ages:
Talk like a human being and behave like a human animal.

Age of Enlightenment:
Talk like a human being and behave like a human being.

Philosopher Queen Sharon Esther Lampert

God Talks to Me: A Working Definition of God

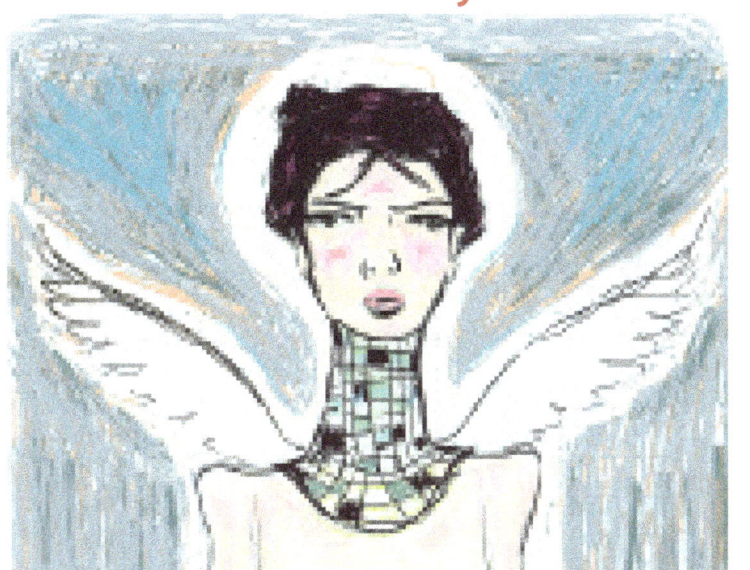

PHYSICAL WORLD
Read My Book
GOD OF WHAT?
11 Esoteric Laws
of Inextricability
Is Life a Gift or a Punishment?

Philosopher Queen
Sharon Esther Lampert

METAPHYSICAL WORLD
Read My Book
UNLEASH THE CREATOR THE GOD WITHIN:
10 Esoteric Laws of Genius and Creativity

Prodigy Queen
Sharon Esther Lampert

And God said:
Go to Work! The Scientific Revolution!
Physical World at Work!

Evolution! Ecosystems! Epigenetics! Extinction!
Marvelous Workers! Biodiversity!
Magnificent Work! 11 Esoteric Laws of Inextricability!

Metaphysical World at Work!

Unconscious to Conscious
Irrational to Rational
(SAVAGE) Ignorance to Knowledge to Wisdom (SAGE)
Innovation & Disruption
Marvelous Workers! Homosapiens!
Magnificent Work! 10 Esoteric Laws of Genius & Creativity!
Work a Miracle! Protect My Elephants from Psychopath Poachers!

26

Dear God,
Does the Universe have a Beginning and a End? What Came First: Chicken or Egg?

'The Best Possible Explanation Is the Simplest!"
— William Ockham "Ochham's Razer"

God Talks to Me: A Working Definition of God

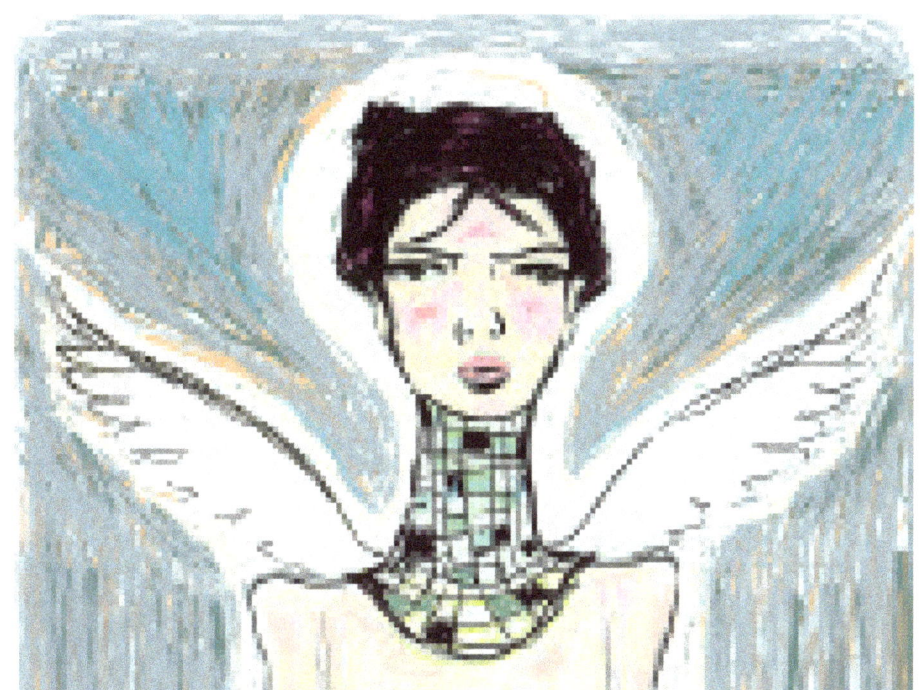

And God said: Go to Work!
BE THE CENTER OF YOUR OWN UNIVERSE!
A CIRCLE HAS NO BEGINNING AND NO END
Circles: Sun, Moon, Planets, Womb, Egg, and Head
Circles: Basketball, Volleyball, Baseball, Tennis Ball, Golf Ball
Work a Miracle! There Are Three Games in Life!
Game 1. WIN:WIN   Collaboration! e.g., Orchestra
Game 2. WIN:LOSE   Competition! e.g., Sports
Game 3. LOSE:LOSE   EVIL e.g., Suicide Bombers!
Marvelous Work! Practice Good Sportsmanship!

27

Dear God,
Do You Run the World or Does the World Run Itself?

"You've always had the power my dear, you just had to learn it for yourself!"

— Glinda, The Good Witch of the North, Wizard of Oz

God Talks to Me: A Working Definition of God

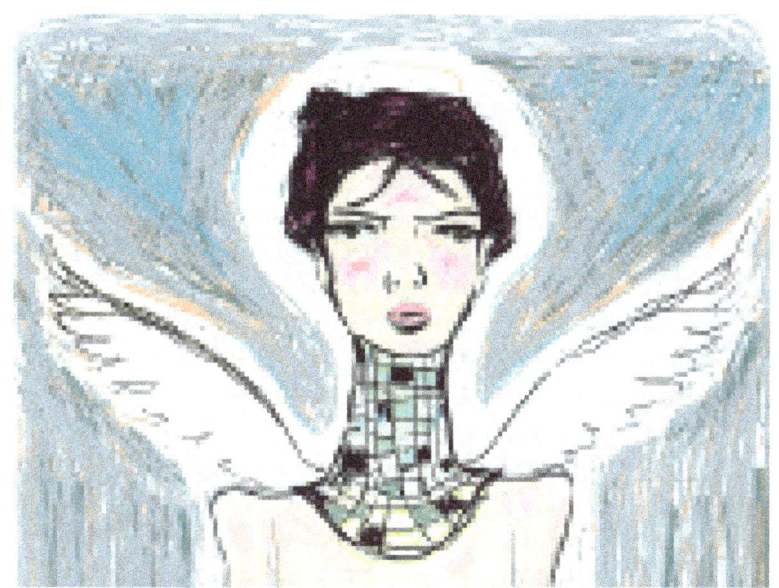

And God said:
THE QUEEN HAS ARRIVED!
Mighty Workers! THE FUTURE IS FEMALE!
Your Vagina Is the Gatekeeper!
Women Have All the Power and Will to Run the Home, Office, and the World!
Mighty Worker! Prime Minister Jacinda Ardern
Magnificent Work! Breaking News Report!
New Zealand Bans All Military Assault Weapons!
Work a Miracle! Female Genital Mutilation Is a Crime!

28

Dear God,

When will nations beat their swords into plowshares, and spears into pruning hooks? Nation shall not lift up sword against nation, neither shall they learn war any more!

—Isaiah 2:4

"Good People, Nothing Is a Problem; Bad People Everything Is a Problem!"
—Philosopher Queen Sharon Esther Lampert

God Talks to Me: A **Working** Definition of God

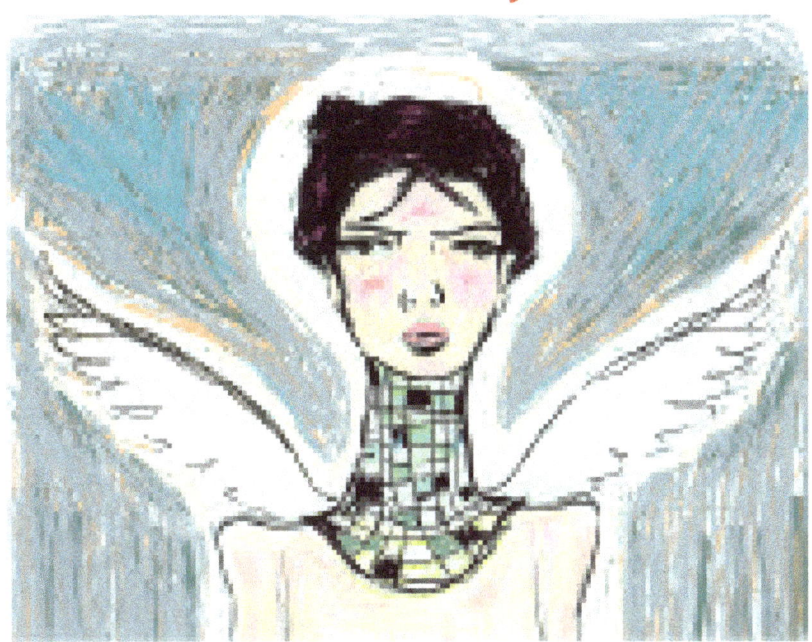

And God said: Failure by Design
Go to Work! GENETICS: DNA, Disorders, and Defects
All EVIL IS JUSTIFIED!
Mother Nature: Poisonous Plants, Poisonous Snakes, and Poisonous Psychopaths

Warmongers, Gangs, Islamic—Jihadist Terrorists, Bogeyman, and Devil

Mass Murderers: School Shooters and Serial Killers

Anti—Social Personality Disorders: Naysayers, Haters, Killjoys, Sourpusses, Wet Blankets, Bullies, and Curmudgeons!

Double Whammy: Nasty Nature! & Nasty Nurture!

Work Miracles! "CRISPR" Genome Editing Technology
(Clustered Regularly Interspaced Short Palindromic Repeats, Nobel Prize 2020)

What Is the Greatest Lie Ever Told in The Name of God?

Sharon Esther Lampert

Concentration Camps: 1939-1945
- Arbeitsdorf
- Auschwitz
- Bergen-Belsen
- Buchenwald
- Dachau
- Flossenbürg
- Gross-Rosen
- Herzogenbusch
- Hinzert
- Kaiserwald
- Kauen
- Kraków-Płaszów
- Majdanek
- Mauthausen
- Mittelbau-Dora
- Natzweiler-Struthof
- Neuengamme
- Niederhagen
- Ravensbrück
- Sachsenhausen
- Stutth
- Vaivara
- Warsaw

Q. Why is the Death of Jesus Good for Christians and Bad for Jews?

Death of Jesus = Christians Get Eternal Life
Deicide = Jews Get 23 Centuries of Persecution
Jesus: Born a Jew & Died a Jew
Early Christians Are Jews
Read Book by Roman Catholic Priest Edward Flannery
"The Anguish of the Jews: Twenty-Three Centuries of Antisemitism"

29

"When You're Jewish, There Is No Such Thing as Too Much Drama!"
—Prophet Sharon Esther Lampert
Princess Kadimah
8TH Prophetess of Israel

Auschwitz Tattoo
August 10, 1944
Susan Rosza —Hungary
A/B20770

Dear God, What About Genocide?

And 23 Centuries of Persecution

"I shall not remain insignificant! I shall work in the world and for mankind! Be kind and have courage."
Annelies Marie "Anne" Frank, Age 15
Died 1945, Bergen–Belsen Concentration Camp, Germany

Wherever Jews Go, Grass Grows!
Wherever Israelis Go, Gardens Grow!
And Gorgeous Glamour Girls! — Gal Gadot

German Sign Posted on Concentration Camp "ARBET MACHES FRIE"– "Work Makes One Free" Enslaved Jews Who Woorked Escaped Gas Chamber! 6 Million Murdered—6000 Gassed Daily

Note: Most Famous Beautiful Women in the World Converted to Judaism: Elizabeth Taylor, Marilyn Monroe, and Ivanka Trump

God Talks to Me: A Working Definition of God

59

13 Israeli Nobel Prizes

1966
Shmuel Yosef Agnon
Literature

1978
Menachem Begin
Peace: Egypt

1994
Shimon Peres & Yitzhak Rabin
Peace: Oslo Accords

2002
Daniel Kahneman
Economics

2004
Aaron Ciechanover & Avram Hershko
Chemistry

2005
Robert Auman
Economics

2009
Ada Yonath (WOMAN)
Chemistry

2011
Dan Shechtman
Chemistry

2013
Michael Levitt & Arieh Warshel
Chemistry

2021
Joshua David Angrist
Economics

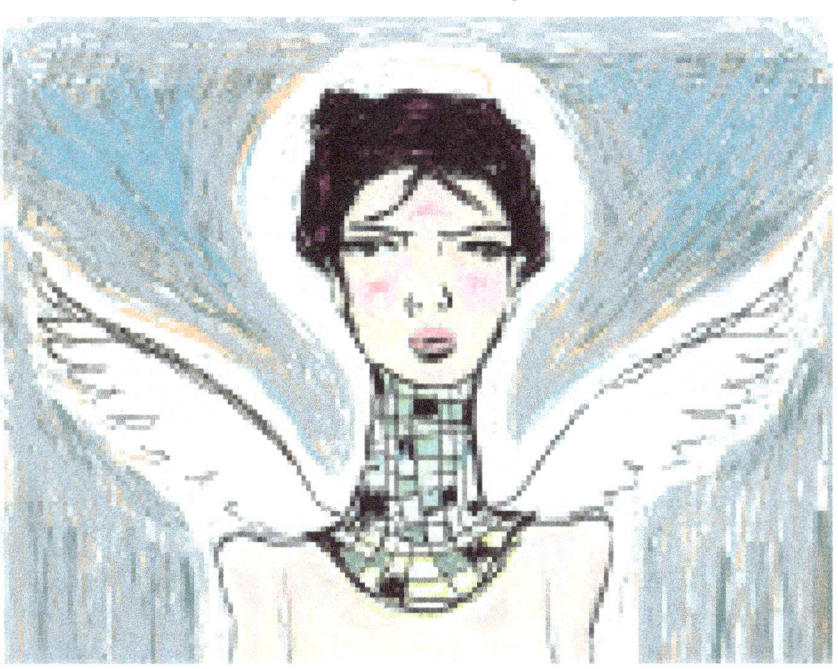

13 Olympic Medals—3 Gold!

"For you are a holy people to the Lord your God; the Lord your God has chosen you to be a people for his own possession out of all the peoples who are on the face of the earth."
—**Deuteronomy 7:6**

Japan's Kyoto Prize
23% Jewish Recipients

US Medal of Science
38% Jewish Recipients

French Academy of Science
48% Jewish Recipients

And God said to ISRAEL

Go to Work! What About a Start Up in an Arid Desert?
Good Work! Drip Irrigation Technology!
Great Works: Jews Are Less Than 1% of the Human Population and 22% of 5 Nobel Prizes! 210 Nobel Prizes! (2022)
Chemistry (36), Literature (16), Physics (56), Economics (35), Physiology or Medicine (58), and Peace (9)
13 Israelis Won the Nobel Prize!
Work Miracles! Sheep to Slaughter to Lions & Light of the World!
May 14, 1948 – HAPPY 75th BIRTHDAY – May 14, 2023
Jewish New Year 5784 (2023)

30
Dear God, What is the Meaning of Life?
Make My Life Make Sense!

"Insanity is the First Law of Nature" Philosopher Queen Sharon Esther Lampert

"There Is No LIFE on Planet Earth: There Is Only a State of LIFELESSNESS!"
The Universe Is Organized by LAWS OF INEXTRICABILITY.
—Philosopher Queen Sharon Esther Lampert

God Talks to Me: A Working Definition of God

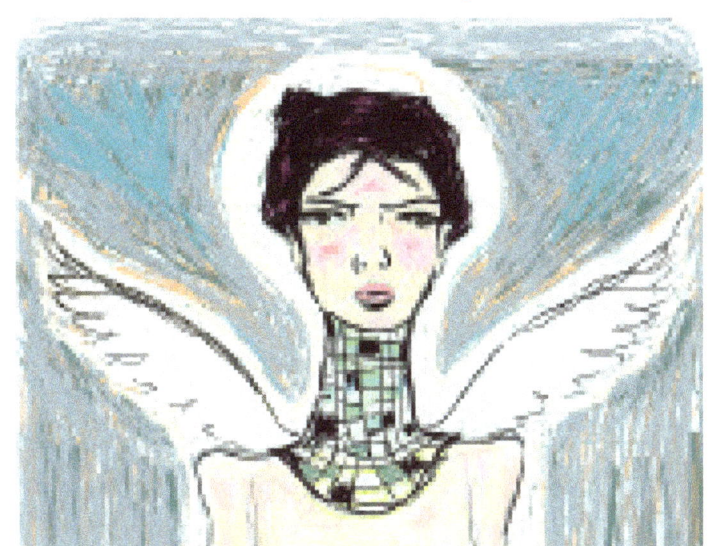

Read My Book:
"Temporary Insanity: We Are Building Our Lives on a Sand Trap"
— Written in Letter S

—Prodigy
Sharon Esther Lampert

The Awesome Art of Alliteration Using One Letter of the Alphabet

And God said: So Simple!
Go to Work! Make Life Make Sense!

Survival = Struggle, Stress, Sacrifice, and Suffering (e.g., Satan)
School of Students: Subjects, Study, Study Skills, School Supplies and Skill Sets
Service to Society & Slavery & Sleep for Stamina & Strength!
Society of Saints & Sinners: Smart%, Stupid% & Sick% Socialization: Savage to Sage!
SUCCESS STRATEGY: Stipulation of Stress, Struggle, Sacrifice and Suffering!
Souls Supplicate with Scripture, Songs, and Sermons to a Savior for SALVATION!
Search for a Sanctuary of Sacred Spaces of Silence, Stillness, Solitude & Serenity!
Spinning Sphere — Sun is a Star in Space in Solar System of Starlight and Satellites!
Seek Shelter, Safety, and Security from Storms — Sanity & InSanity
#STAYSTRONG Sickness, Sorrow, Suffering & SAND TRAP!
SEX Starts Sequence from Stratch — Survival to Sand Trap!
Surrender to the System — Sunrise to Sunset — Survival to Sand Trap!
See Savior in Signs & Symbols!

31

Dear God, Is Life a Gift or a Punishment?

Billions of People Have Lived and Died on Planet Earth.
Why Is Planet Earth Still a Torture Chamber of Unspeakable Horrors?

99.9% of People Do Not Have to Look
Outside Their Own Families to Find Hatred!

EVIL IS EVERYWHERE
EPOCH, ERA, EON, AND ETERNITY

—Philosopher Queen Sharon Esther Lampert

God Talks to Me: A Working Definition of God

Read My Book:
THERAPY
— Written in Letter T

Test
Tragedy
Trauma
Tears
Time

Philosopher Queen
Sharon Esther Lampert

The Awesome Art
of Alliteration
Using One Letter
of the Alphabet

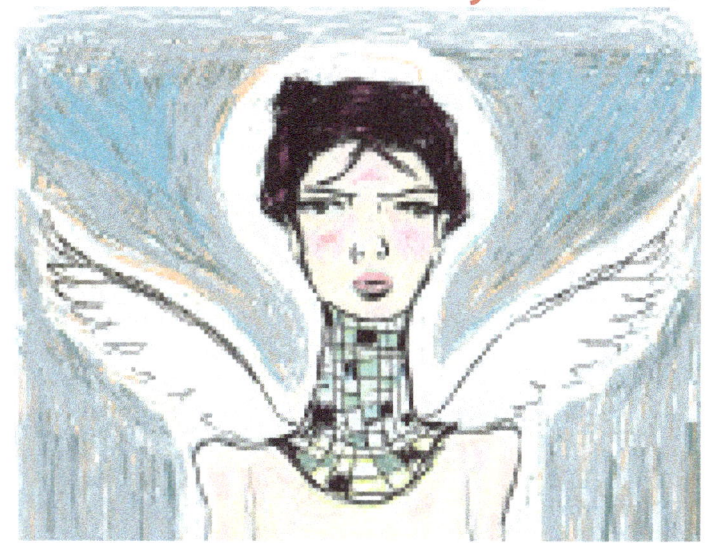

And God said:
Measure the Pain! Measure the Pleasure!
Go to Work! Count Your Smiles!
Go to Work! Count Your Tears!
Every Day, You Will Take a Test!
What Test Did You Take Today?

Mighty Workers! Psychiatrists! Therapists! Counselors! Healers! Indian Gurus!

Life is Temporary Insanity of Dizzy Daydreams and Crazy Nightmares!

Play the Cards You Have! Listen to Your Inner Voice! Stay in Your Own Lane!

Find Your Passion, Fulfill Your Potential, and Find Your Place in the World!

Time Cannot Be Saved! You Are Always Spending Your Time! Waste Not!

Put LOVE into Everything You Do!

Leave a Legacy!

32

Dear God, Why Do We Suffer Before We Die?

"What if my whole life has been wrong?"
"The Death of Ivan Ilyich" by Leo Tolstoy

God Talks to Me: A Working Definition of God

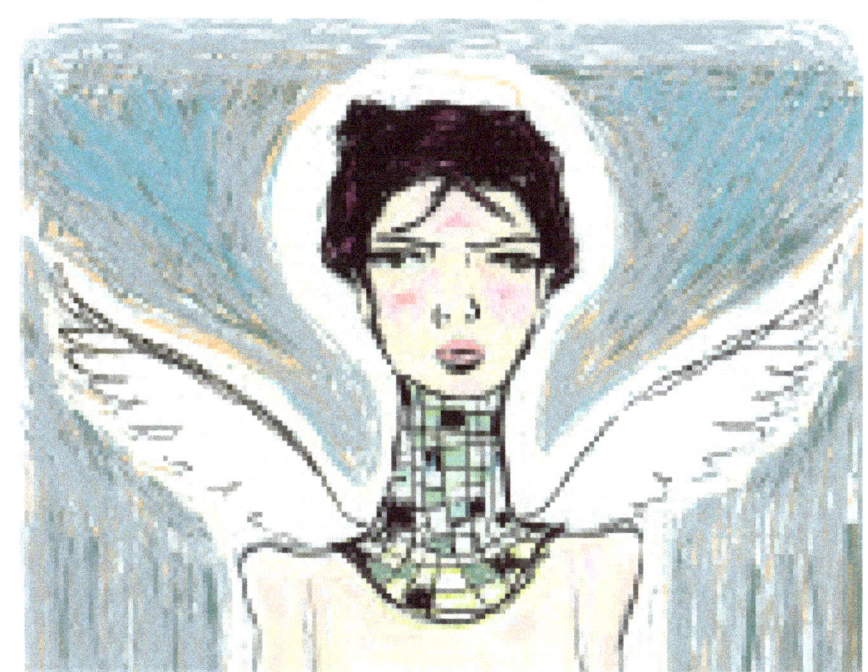

And God said:
Go to Work! Document Your Life!
Memories Fade! You Will Not Be Able to Remember Having Lived a Life!
Suffering Began on the Day You Were Born
EVERY DAY IS A FIGHT FOR SURVIVAL!
STRESS, STRUGGLE, SACRIFICE, AND SUFFERING
You Are Born Without Your Consent
You Can Exercise FREE WILL and Leave at Any Time:
Simply Skip a Few Meals or Dramatically by Suicide
Meaningful Work! Death with Dignity!

33

Dear God,

Is There One or Many Metaphysical Gods?
Are There Messengers of God?
Prophets? Angels? Holy Spirits? Saints?
Son of God? Ancestor Worship?
Yoda and The Force?

"May The Force Be With You!"

JEDI Sharon Esther Lampert

God Talks to Me: A Working Definition of God

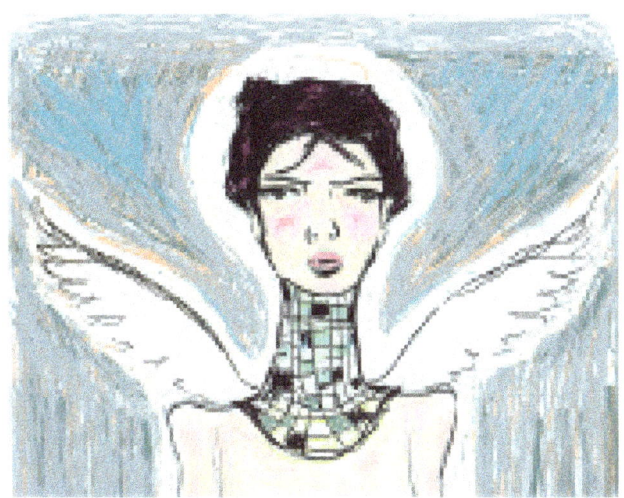

And God said:
Go to Work! Take My God Quiz!
For Centuries, Believers of All Faiths, Recite One Prayer:
"Help Me, Heal Me, and Protect Me from Harm!"

Take My God Quiz?
Q. Which Statement is True?
  a. God Will Protect Me!
  b. God Helps Those Who Help Themselves!
  c. God Does Not Exist!

Meaningful Work!   Follow Your Own Internal GPS!
Marvelous Work!   Follow Your Bliss!
Magnificent Work! Live Your Truth!

The correct answer is b. God Helps Those Who Help Themselves! God It? Good!
God Can Only Do for You What God Can Do Through You!

Sharon Esther left a note in Israel's Wailing Wall:

"Dear God,
I am not asking for help.
I am offering to be of help.
I am at your service!"

Sharon Esther Lampert, Age 16

Sharon Esther Lampert

34

Dear God,

What's Going on God?
What's Doing God?
World Peace?

"When God sees you doing your part, developing what she has given you, then she will do her part, and open doors that no one can shut!"
—Revelation 3:8

Moses Has 10 Commandments. You Have 22 Commandments!
YOU HAD TO OUTDO MOSES!
—Joel Rappelfeld

www.WORLD PEACE EQUATION.com

God Talks to Me: A Working Definition of God

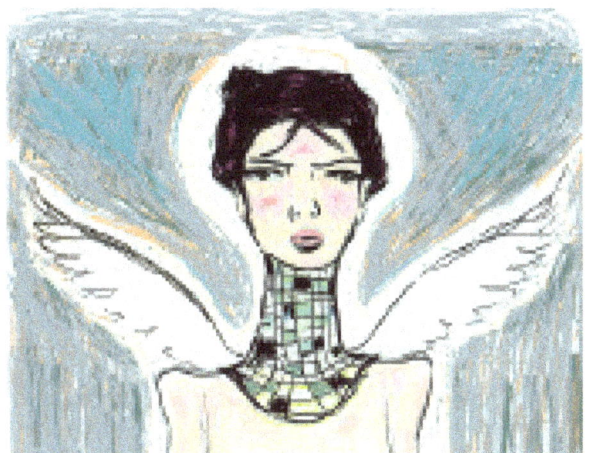

FAN MAIL

"Dear Princess Kadimah, 8TH Prophetess of Israel, I was reading your 22 Commandments. Reminds me of a book I recently read by Rabbi Donniel, "Putting God Second." In defense from God Intoxication we must even hold religion accountable to basic ethical principles."
—Robert

Read My Book
THE 22 COMMANDMENTS
Princess Kadimah
8TH Prophetess of Israel
Sharon Esther Lampert

A Universal
Moral Compass
For All People
For All Religions
For All Time

And God said: Go to Work!
THE 22 COMMANDMENTS
All You Will Ever Need to Know About God

1. LIFE Over Death
2. STRENGTH Over Weakness
3. DEED Over Sin
4. LOVE Over Hatred
5. TRUTH Over Lie
6. COURAGE Over Fear
7. OPTIMISM Over Pessimism
8. SHARING Over Selfishness
9. PRAISE Over Criticism
10. LOYALTY Over Abandonment
11. RESPONSIBILITY Over Blame
12. GRATITUDE Over Envy
13. REWARD Over Punishment
14. ALLIES Over Enemies
15. CREATION Over Destruction
16. EDUCATION Over Ignorance
17. COOPERATION Over Competition
18. FREEDOM Over Oppression
19. COMPASSION Over Indifference
20. FORGIVENESS Over Revenge
21. PEACE Over War
22. JOY Over Suffering

By Sharon Esther Lampert, Princess Kadimah, 8TH Prophetess of Israel

35

Dear God, What is LOVE?

Q. Why Is the Person You Love and Married the Same Person You Hate and Divorced?

Read My Book: "CUPID" — Written in Letter C
"Connection! Chemistry! Communication! Compatibility! Companionship! Commitment! Consummation!"
—Prodigy Sharon Esther Lampert

God Talks to Me: A Working Definition of God

71

Read My Book:
"LOVE YOU MORE THAN YESTERDAY"
14 Relationship Strategies for Happily Ever After!

—Prodigy
Sharon Esther Lampert

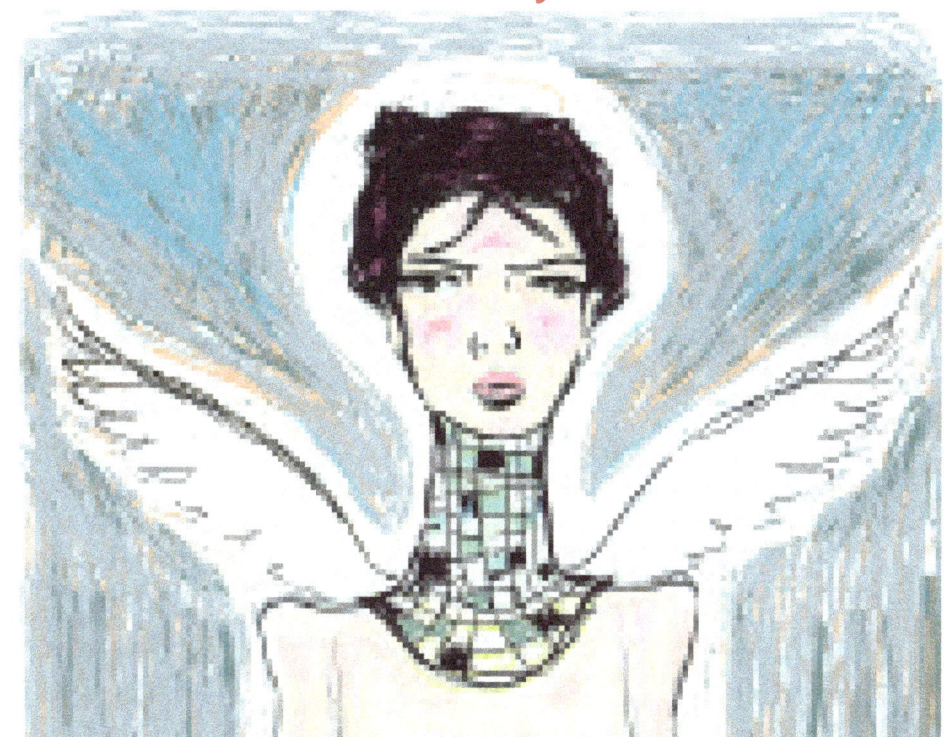

And God said: Go to Work!
You Don't Find LOVE; You Create LOVE
Practice Respect, Understanding, Empathy, Kindness, and Tolerance
TRUE LOVE IS UNCONDITIONAL LOVE!
Unconditional Love Is Real — But Rare! — Get a Loyal Pet!
You Can Never Know Another Person!
All People Help You with Their Strengths & Hurt You with Their Weaknesses!
Practice SelfLOVE: Selfcare Is Not Selfish!
The Most Important Relationship Is the One You Have with Yourself!
Love from Outside of Yourself Is Extra: BONUS LOVE!

36

Dear God,

What's Up with Heaven or Down with Hell,
and Reincarnation or Transmigration of the Soul?
Is There a Day of Judgment: Paradise or Purgatory?
In other words: **Is My Soul Immortal?**

The State of Your Soul

5 Out of 5 People Suffer Mental Health Distress
1 Out of 5 Suffer from an Undiagnosed Mental Disorder (genetic defect)
1 Out of 10 Is a Functional Psychotic (poisonous snake)
1 Out of 25 Is a Psychopath (poisonous snake)

Philosopher Queen Sharon Lampert

God Talks to Me: A Working Definition of God

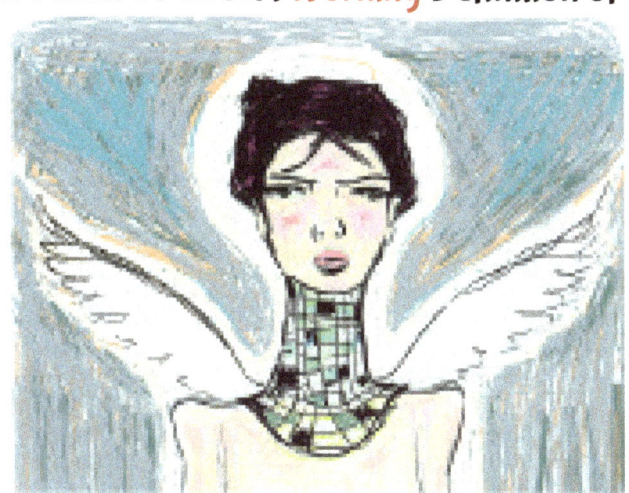

And God said:
Go to Work! Work Like Hell!
Everything Goes Wrong Before It Goes Right!
You Are Born Unconscious, Irrational, and Ignorant!
You Are a Work in Progress! Mind, Body, and Soul!
You Cannot Right the Wrongs of the Past!
Work a Miracle! Every Day Is a Fresh Start!
Every Day Is a New Possibility to Get It Right!

Your SEED Not Your SOUL Is Immortal
DNA (SEED) Is Immortal, and Is Passed Down
from One Generation to the Next
Your SOUL is Fragile and Finite, BUT(BIG BUT)
Every SOUL Is a One-of-a Kind Fingerprint!
Fragile: One Wrong Move — Game Over!
Finite: Time Cannot be Saved — Waste Not!
Fingerprint: Leave an Indelible Legacy!

37

Dear God, Is there LIFE after DEATH?

God Talks to Me: A Working Definition of God

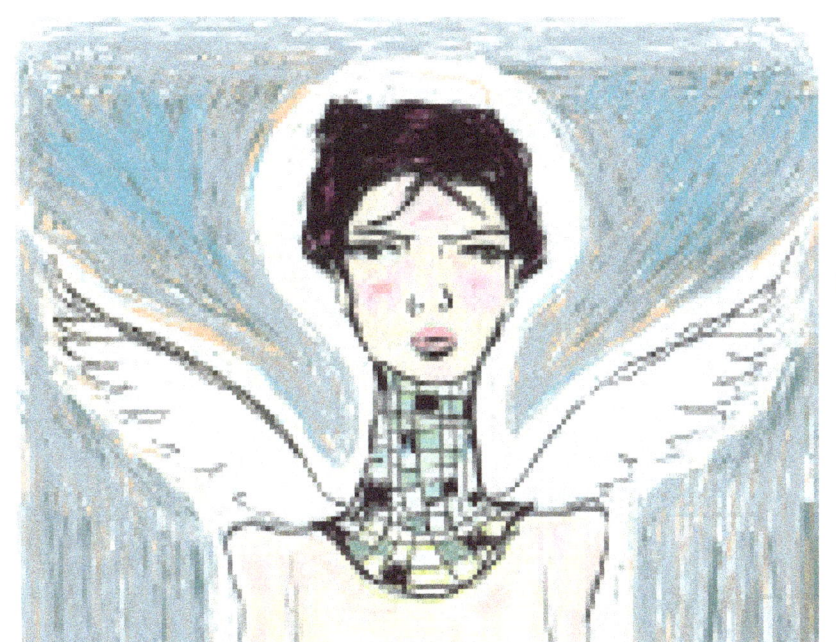

BE ART
ART IS SMART
ART IS OF THE HEART
MAKE ART NOT WAR
YOU ARE BORN FOR GREATNESS
YOU ARE A MASTERPIECE

Sharon Esther Lampert
Gift Shop: artheart.store

And God said:
Go to Work! The Digital Revolution

BE ART! You Are Born for Greatness! You Are a Masterpiece!

Great Works! You will live forever in still-life photography & walkie-talkie videos! ART IS SMART! ART IS OF THE HEART! MAKE ART NOT WAR!

Work Movie Magic! Create a YOUTUBE channel featuring your life: Your mother's excruciatingly painful birth; Your cute childhood years of learning how to walk, talk, and share your toys; Your raging hormonal teen years of identity angst; Your adult years of domestic-family dysfunction; and your senior years of crabby, cranky, and cursing the day you were born into a cruel world!

38

Dear God,
I worked like a DOG!
I have bags under my eyes,
wrinkles on my face,
my knees creek, and
my bones ache!

"Talent hits a target no one else can hit— Genius hits a target no one else can see!"
– Arthur Schopenhauer

God Talks to Me: A Working Definition of God

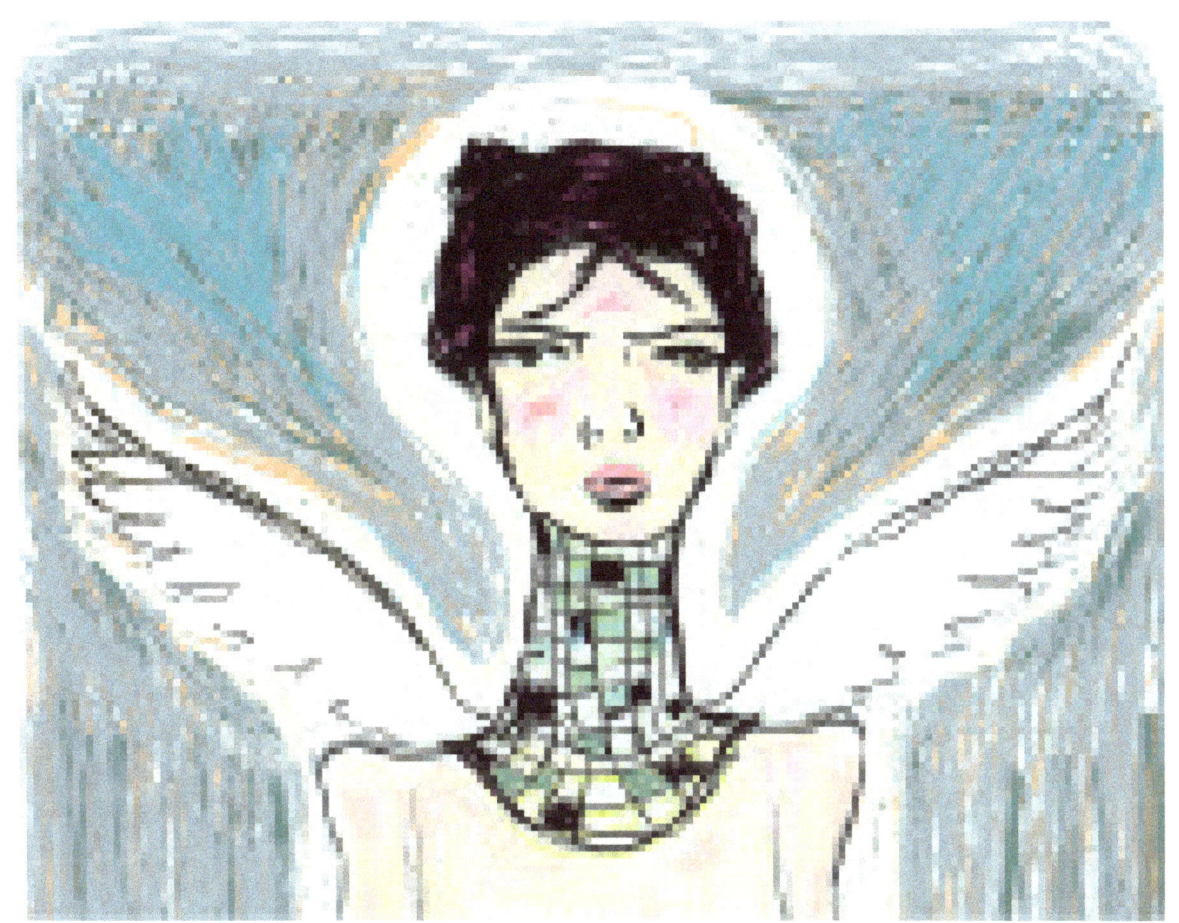

And God said:
Go to Work! Dig a Grave, a Deep Hole Under the Ground. It's Time to Die!
DOG Spelled Backward Is GOD!

39
Do you hear the voice of God ringing in your ears too?

Go to Work!

God Talks to Me!
God Talks to You!
God Talks to Everyone!

Sharon Esther Lampert
Prophet, Philosopher Queen, Prodigy Poet, Peacemaker, Princess & Pea, PHOTON & Paladin of Education, Performer, Player, President, Publisher, Producer, Phoenix, and PINUP!
Princess Kadimah 8TH Prophetess of Israel

Passion, Purpose, Patience, Positivity, Perserverance, Productivity, Progress, Power, Prosperity, Peace

God Talks to Me: A Working Definition of God

Read My Book:
POWER
— Written in Letter P

Passion
Purpose
Plan in Place on Paper
Patience
Perseverance
Progress

Prodigy
Sharon Esther Lampert

The Awesome Art
of Alliteration
Using One Letter
of the Alphabet

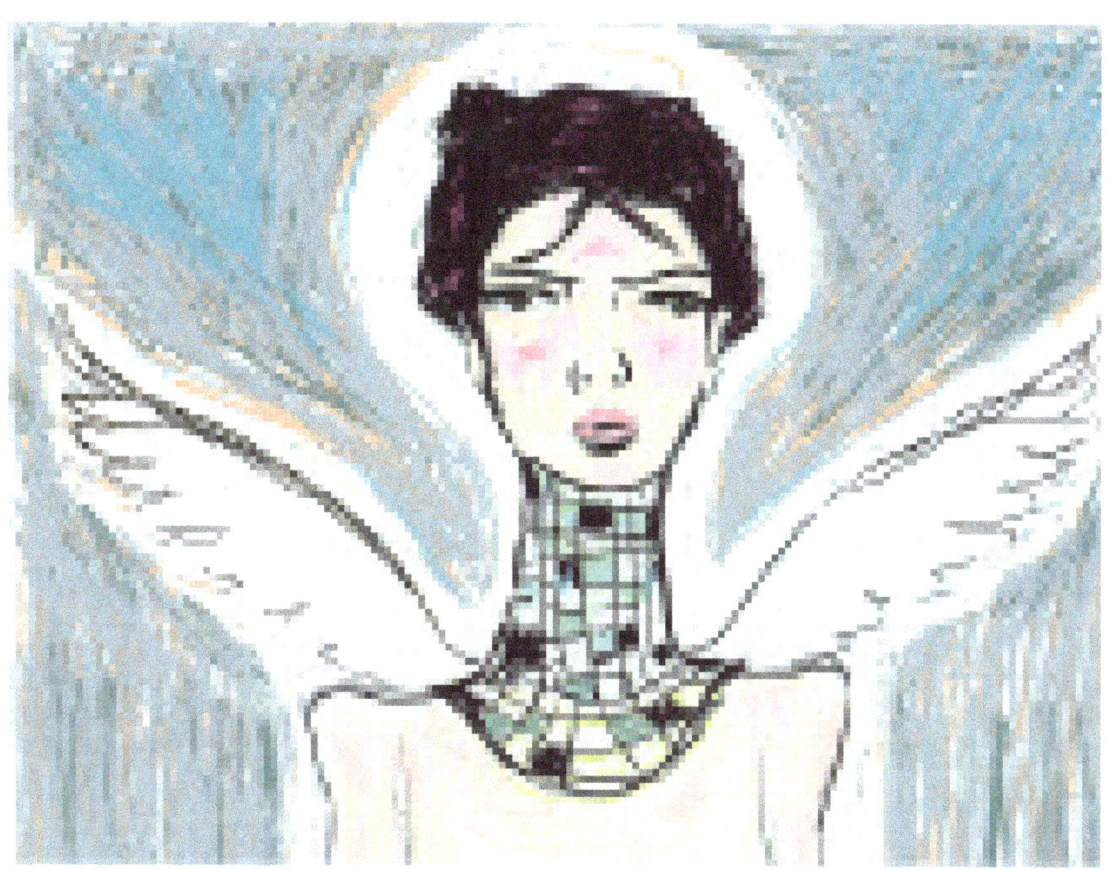

And God said: Go to Work!
To Every Living Being Flying in the Sky, Swimming in the Sea, and Crawling or Walking on Dry Land! **GOD IS GO! DO!**

40

Dear God,

Yes! I can hear you talk to me!
GOD IS GO! DO!
God Can Only Do For You What God Can Do Through You!

Just two more questions — maybe five?????
When I pray to you, do you hear me?
7.9 billion people pray to you — some 5X a day — do you hear them?

"Prayer is when you speak and God listens, and meditation is when God speaks and you listen."
—Dr. Sukhraj Dhillon

Gift Shop: GodIsGoDo.com

God Talks to Me: A Working Definition of God

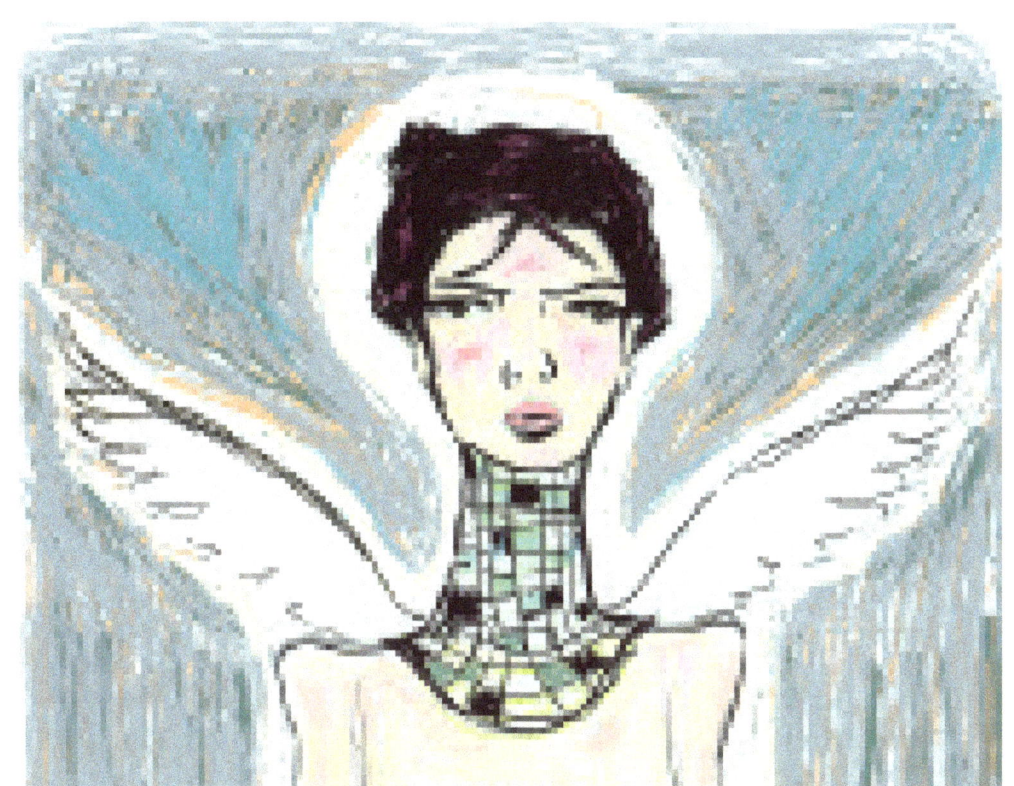

And God said to 4000+ Religions
Don't Wish for It! Work for It!
Fight to Live! Live to Fight! Born to Die!
The Harder You Work, the Luckier You Get!
My Temple and Religion Are: Good Works!
Got It! Good! Get to Work!
Early is On Time! On Time is Late! Late is Unacceptable!

There Are No Believers:
There Are Make-Believers
and Non-Believers!

Philosopher Queen
Sharon Lampert

41

Dear God, Do You Even Exist?

"God Is Not Physics: The Laws of the Universe!
God is Metaphysics: Beyond the Scope of Scientific Inquiry!
There Is a Physical and Metaphysical Universe!
God Is an Invisible and Intangible Entity Like Our Mind, Thoughts, and Ideas.
God Can Only Do For You, What God Can Do Through You!"

Sharon Esther Lampert, Princess Kadimah, 8TH Prophetess of Israel

God Talks to Me: A Working Definition of God

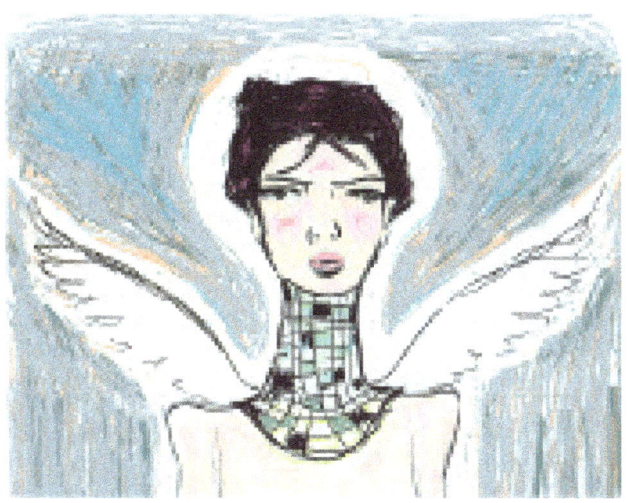

Read My Book
GOD OF WHAT?
11 Esoteric Laws
of Inextricability
Is Life a Gift or a Punishment?

Philosopher Queen
Sharon Esther Lampert

Read My Book
UNLEASH THE CREATOR THE GOD WITHIN:
10 Esoteric Laws of Genius and Creativity

Prodigy Queen
Sharon Esther Lampert

And God said:
Go to Work! Unleash The Creator The God Within!
God Can Only Do For You, What God Can Do Through You!
Who Are You?
To Ask Me!
Who It Is?
That I Am!

Do You Even Exist?
Here Today! Gone Tomorrow!

42

Dear God, What happens when you dress up Albert Einstein as Marilyn Monroe?

NO FAKES! NO FAT! NO FLUFF! NO FILLER! NO FLOPS! NO FUDGE! NO F-BOMB!

God Talks to Me: A Working Definition of God

About the Author

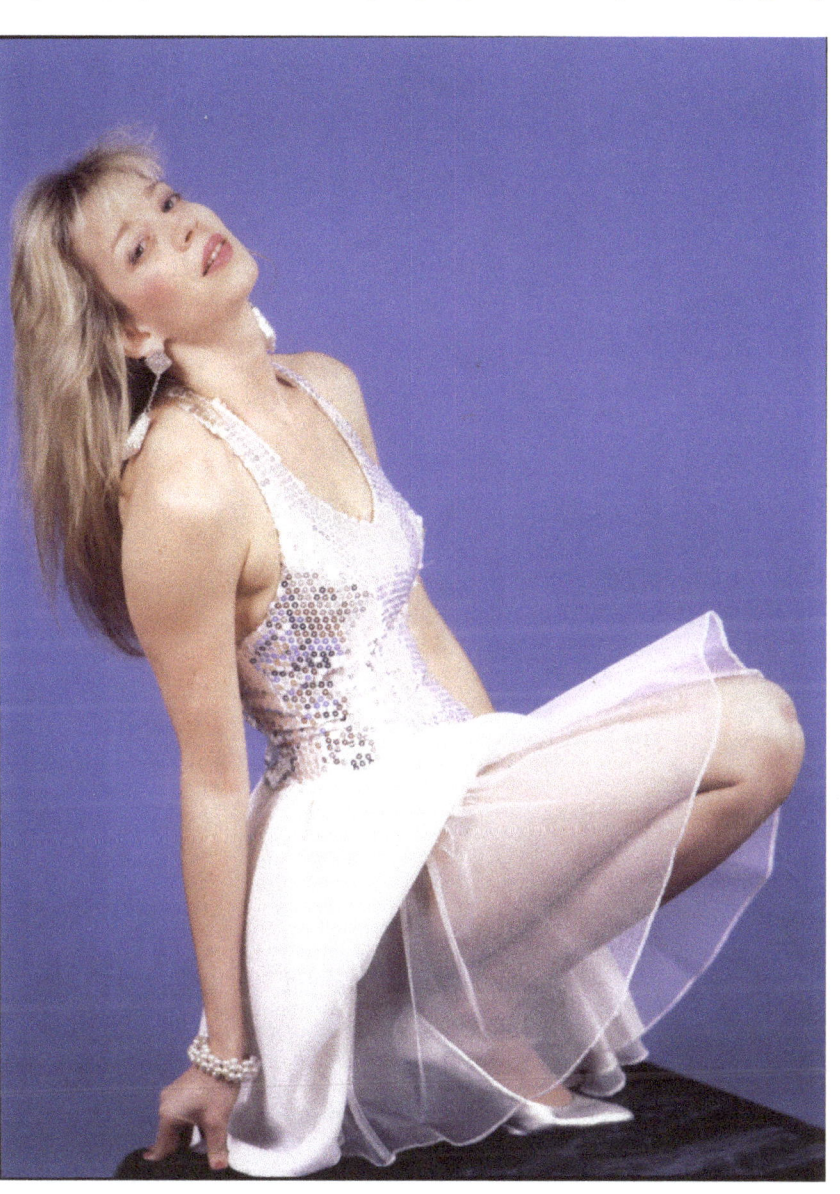

Sharon Esther Lampert

MYLIFE Is an OPENBOOK, to KNOWME Is to README

**1.
PRODIGY**
10 Esoteric Laws of Genius & Creativity

**2.
POET**
The Greatest Poems Ever Written on Extraordinary World Events

**3.
PHILOSOPHER**
TEMPORARY INSANITY Make Life Make Sense
—Written in Letter S

CUPID
Language of Love
—Written in Letter C

**4.
PROPHET**
22 COMMANDMENTS
A Universal Moral Compass For All People

GOD TALKS TO ME
A WORKING DEFINITION OF GOD
GOD IS GO! DO!

**5.
PHOTON &
PALADIN OF EDUCATION**
SMARTGRADES BRAIN POWER REVOLUTION

**6.
PINUP**
SEXIEST CREATIVE GENIUS IN HUMAN HISTORY

43

Dear God, What happens when you dress down Albert Einstein as Marilyn Monroe?

Voluptuous, Vivacious, Valiant, Vanguard, and V.E.S.S.E.L.

God Talks to Me: A Working Definition of God

About the Author

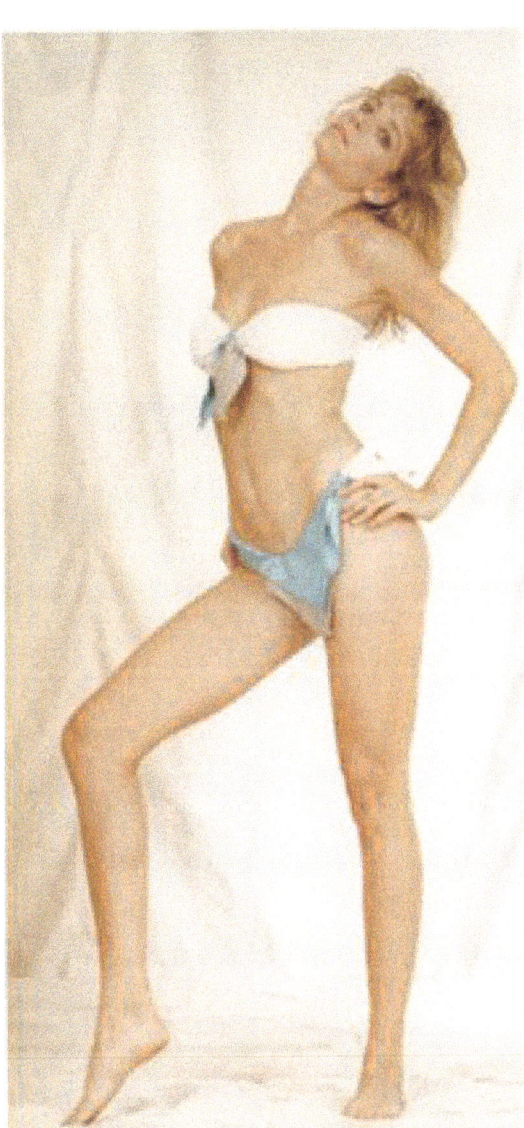

Sharon Esther Lampert

MYLIFE Is an OPENBOOK, to KNOWME Is to README

1.
PRODIGY
10 Esoteric Laws of Genius & Creativity

2.
POET
The Greatest Poems Ever Written on Extraordinary World Events

3.
PHILOSOPHER
TEMPORARY INSANITY Make Life Make Sense
—Written in Letter S

CUPID
Language of Love
—Written in Letter C

4.
PROPHET
22 COMMANDMENTS
A Universal Moral Compass For All People

GOD TALKS TO ME
A WORKING DEFINITION OF GOD
GOD IS GO! DO!

5.
**PHOTON &
PALADIN OF EDUCATION**
SMARTGRADES BRAIN POWER REVOLUTION

6.
PINUP
SEXIEST CREATIVE GENIUS IN HUMAN HISTORY

Sexiest Creative Genius in Human History

V.E.S.S.E.L.
Very.
Extra.
Special.
Sharon.
Esther.
Lampert.

PINUP

44

Dear God, Lessons Learned?

God Talks to Me: A Working Definition of God

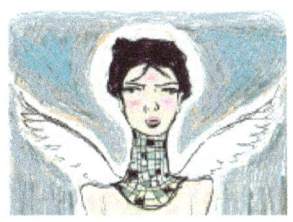

And God said:
Go to Work! Lessons Learned!

1. GOD IS GO DO!

2. God Can Only Do For You What God Can Do Through You! God It!

3. There is a physical universe and a metaphysical universe and they are INEXTRICABLY linked. The universe is organized by LAWS OF INEXTRICABILITY.
   Read My Book: 11 Esoteric Laws of Inextricability (physical world)
   Read My Book: 10 Esoteric Laws of Genius & Creativity (metaphysical world)

4. The metaphysical universe is beyond the scope of scientific inquiry like your mind, thoughts, and ideas (invisible and intagible entities).

5. ROLL THE DICE! In an immoral universe there are 8 probabilities:
   Good goes to (1) good (2) bad (3) good and bad or (4) nothing.
   Bad goes to (1) bad (2) good (3) good and bad or (4) nothing.

6. THE BLIND LEAD THE BLIND: UNCONSCIOUS, IRRATIONAL & IGNORANT
   You are born this way, you will live this way, and you will die this way.

7. There is only one global enemy: IGNORANCE.

8. The Greatest Lie Ever Told in the Name of God Is:
   Q. Why Is the Death of Jesus Good for Christians but Bad for Jews?
      Christians get ETERNAL LIFE and Jews get 23 Centuries of Persecution

9. You are born without your consent — but you can exercise FREE WILL and leave at any time by skipping a few meals or by suicide.

10. Memories fade: You will not be able to remember having lived a life.

Sharon Esther Lampert

About the Author

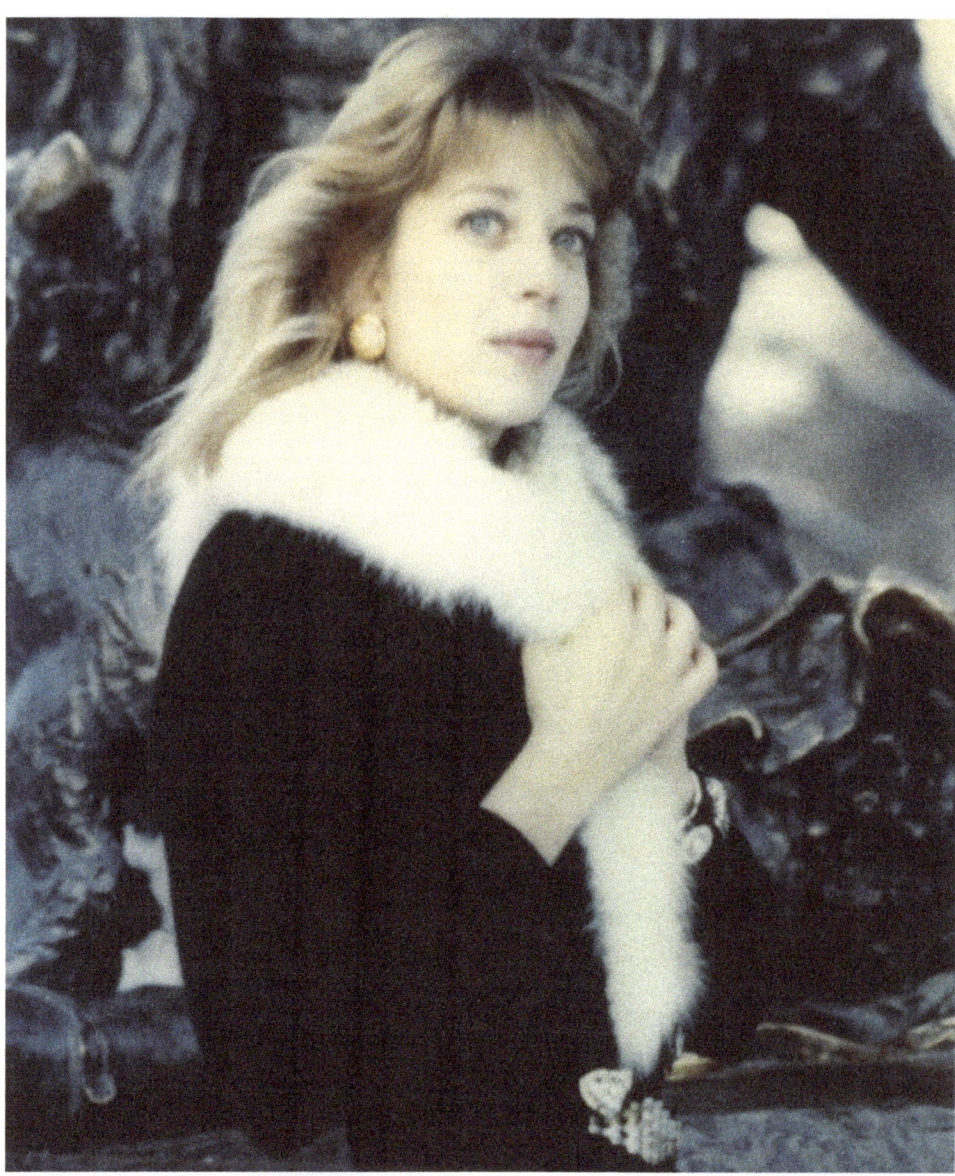

Sharon Esther Lampert

MYLIFE Is an OPENBOOK, to KNOWME Is to READme

1.
PRODIGY
10 Esoteric Laws of Genius & Creativity

2.
POET
The Greatest Poems Ever Written on Extraordinary World Events

3.
PHILOSOPHER
TEMPORARY INSANITY
Make Life Make Sense
—Written in Letter S

CUPID
Language of Love
—Written in Letter C

4.
PROPHET
22 COMMANDMENTS
A Universal Moral Compass For All People

GOD TALKS TO ME
A WORKING DEFINITION OF GOD
GOD IS GO! DO!

5.
PHOTON &
PALADIN OF EDUCATION
SMARTGRADES
BRAIN POWER
REVOLUTION

6.
PINUP
SEXIEST CREATIVE GENIUS IN HUMAN HISTORY

God Talks to Me: A Working Definition of God

At Age 9, my **MOMMY** knew who I was from the **INSIDE OUT!** "My Daughter is a **P**oet, **P**hilosopher, and **T**eacher. **THE QUEEN HAS ARRIVED! Beauty & Brains!**" XOXO **MOMMY**

In 1997, **NYU** honored me at graduation with an **Award** for **Multi-Interdisciplinary Studies** (YouTube videos)

My father's nickname was **BEZALEL**, the artisan in the Bible who created the **Ark of the Covenant**. I inherited the blessing.
EXODUS 31:1-3

SHARON ESTHER LAMPERT
V.E.S.S.E.L. **V**ery. **E**xtra. **S**pecial. **S**haron. **E**sther. **L**ampert.

POET — One of The World's Greatest Poets
The Greatest Poems Ever Written on Extraordinary World Events
WORLD POETRY RECORD
http://famouspoetsandpoems.com/poets.html
18 Books of Poetry

PROPHET — G**O**D IS G**O**! D**O**!
22 COMMANDMENTS: All You Will Ever Need to Know About God
GOD TALKS TO ME: A Working Definition of God

PHILOSOPHER
God of What? **Is Life a Gift or a Punishment?** 10 Absolute Truths
Temporary Insanity — Written in Letter **S**
Sperm Manifesto — 10 Rules for the Road

PEACEMAKER
World Peace Equation.com

PRODIGY
- 10 Esoteric Laws of Genius and Creativity: Unleash the Creator the God Within
- Women Have All the Power — But Have Never Learned How to Use It!
- Silly Little Boys: 40 Rules of Manhood — 14 Global Catastrophes!
- **C**UPID: Language of Love — Written in Letter **C**
- **D**ESTINY: Life By **D**efault or By **D**esign? — Written in Letter **D**
- **T**RAGEDY: Every Day You Have to Take a **T**est — Written in Letter **T**
- **P**UBLISH: The **SECRET SAUCE** of Book Sales — Written in Letter **P**
- My Day, My Dream, My Destiny — Innovation of 7 Time Shifts
- Love You More Than Yesterday (LYMTY) — 14 Relationship Strategies for Happily After Ever
- 10 MIRACLES: What Happens When You FREE Your Mind of NEGATIVITY?

PALADIN OF EDUCATION – SMARTGRADES BRAIN POWER REVOLUTION - 25 BOOKS
- 40 Universal Gold Standards of Education
- 10 SMARTGRADES Learning Tools
- 15 Stepping Stones of Academic Success
- 15 Stumbling Blocks of Academic Failure

Smartgrades.com, PhotonSuperhero.com, EveryDayAnEasyA.com

PHOTON
SUPERHERO OF EDUCATION
www.PhotonSuperhero.com

PINUP
THE SEXIEST CREATIVE GENIUS IN HUMAN HISTORY

PERFORMER
Vocalist: Ashira Orchestra (YOUTUBE Videos)

PLAYER: JOCK
N.Y.U. Women's Varsity Basketball Team, N.Y.C. Marathon, Skiing, Tennis, Weightlifting

---

The **A**wesome **A**rt of **A**lliteration Using One Letter of the **A**lphabet:
1. **C**UPID — **C**
2. Temporary In**s**anity — **S**
3. Secret Sauce — **P**
4. **D**ESTINY — **D**
5. POWER - P
6. **T**HERAPY — **T**
7. What Do Books Do? — E
8. 8 Goalposts of Education — E

Pro**di**gy Sharon Esther writes a whole book in one day or night:
1. CHATTERBOX
2. SCHMALTZY
3. SILLY LITTLE BOYS
4. **C**UPID — **C**
5. **T**EMPORARY IN**S**ANITY — **S**
6. **T**RAGEDY — **T**
7. WIN AT THIN — **A**

EXODUS 31:1-3
1. And the Lord spoke unto Moses, saying,

2. See, I have called by name **BEZALEL** the son of Uri, the son of Hur, of the tribe of Judah:

3. And I have filled him with the spirit of God, in wisdom, and in understanding, and in knowledge, and in all manner of workmanship.

PINUP

Sharon Esther Lampert

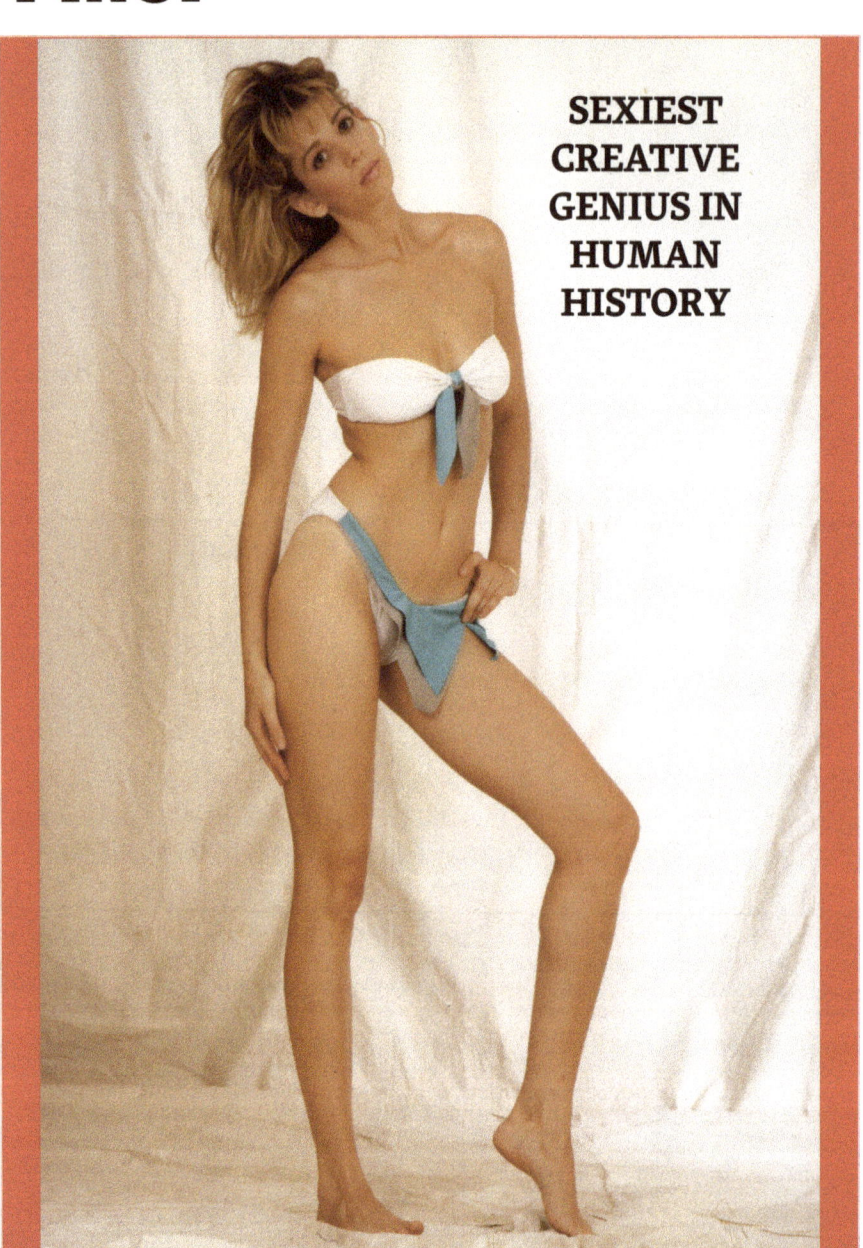

SEXIEST CREATIVE GENIUS IN HUMAN HISTORY

1.
PRODIGY
10 Esoteric Laws of Genius & Creativity

2.
POET
The Greatest Poems Ever Written on Extraordinary World Events

3.
PHILOSOPHER
TEMPORARY INSANITY
Make Life Make Sense
—Written in Letter S

CUPID
Language of Love
—Written in Letter C

4.
PROPHET
22 COMMANDMENTS
A Universal Moral Compass For All People

GOD TALKS TO ME
A WORKING DEFINITION OF GOD
GOD IS GO! DO!

5.
PHOTON & PALADIN OF EDUCATION
SMARTGRADES
BRAIN POWER
REVOLUTION

6.
PINUP
SEXIEST CREATIVE GENIUS IN HUMAN HISTORY

MYLIFE is an OPENBOOK, to KNOWME Is to README

God Talks to Me: A Working Definition of God

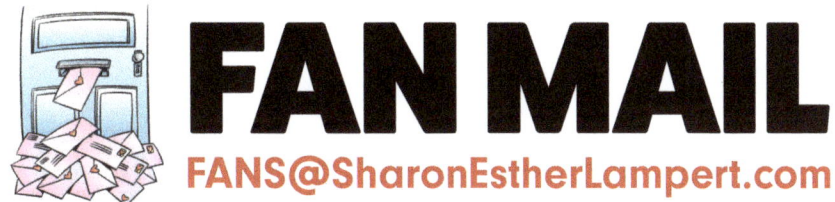

FAN MAIL
FANS@SharonEstherLampert.com

A PHENOMENON...
SHARON ESTHER LAMPERT

Lithe and lovely ... like a fawn.
This lady fascinates me ... from dusk till dawn.
Feminine and comely ... she's beyond belief
A blue-beam from her eyes ... is my soothing relief.

Girlish in her braces ... maidenly in her style
I yearn for her embraces ... and adore her friendly smile.
As tasteful as any artist ... you'll ever see
She's a compendium of class ... from A to Z.

If you'd like to see a figure, that puts Venus to shame
Behold her in a swimsuit, and your passions will aflame.
Ever exuding goodness . . . guided from above
Miss Sharon is the essence, and epitome of Love.

She's the inspiration of sages, and also fools like me
And the most magnificent female, I'm sure I'll ever see.
The nights are now endearing, & never filled with doubt
I sometimes wake up singing, cause it's Sharon . . .
I dream about.

Affectionately, . .
A devoted fan,
—Harry McVeety

Sharon Esther Lampert

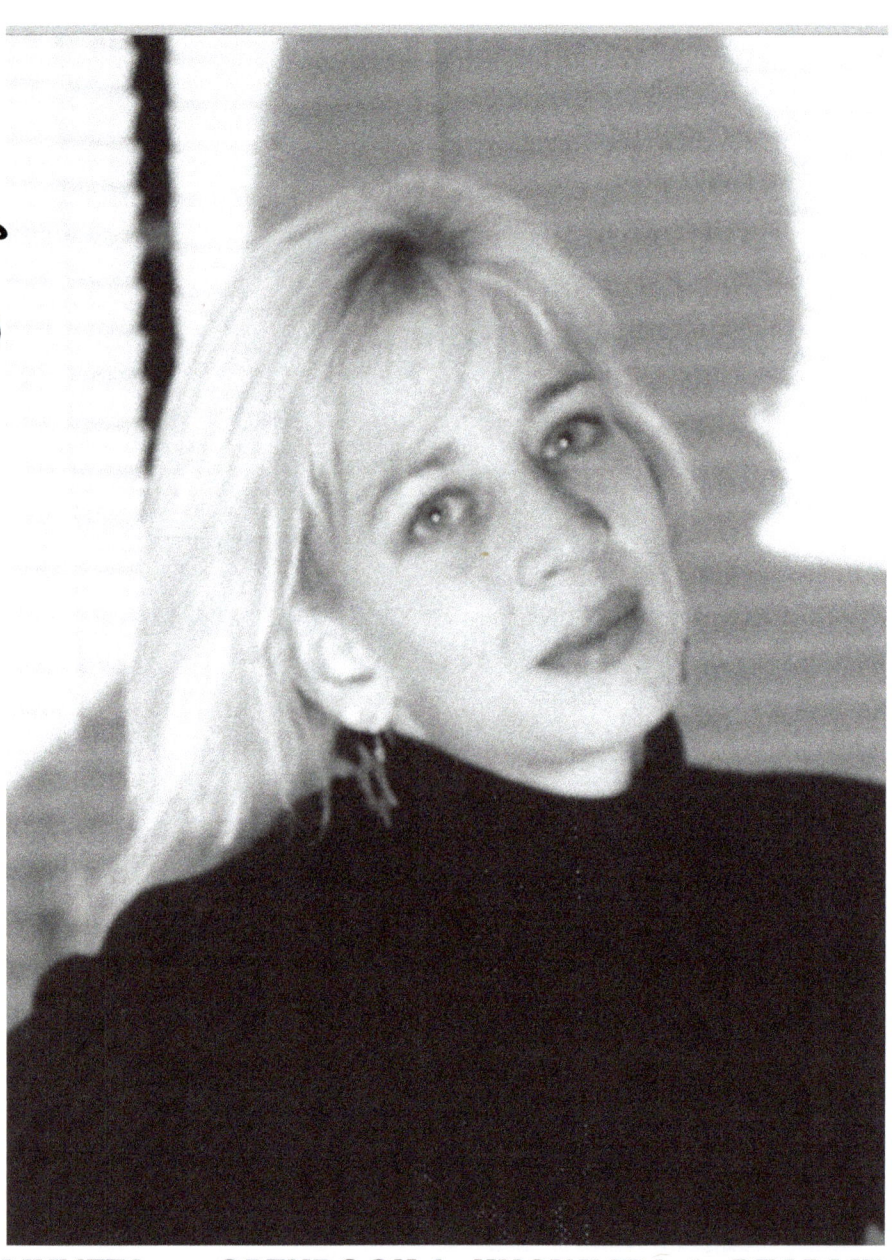

Find The Light and Live In The Light!

Sharon Esther Lampert

Prodigy
Poet
Prophet
Philosopher
Peacemaker
Paladin of
Education
PINUP
PHOTON
Player:Jock
Performer
President
Publisher

MYLIFE is an OPENBOOK, to KNOWME is to README

God Talks to Me: A *Working* Definition of God

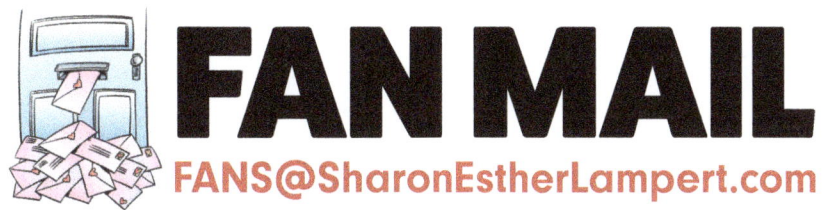

FAN MAIL
FANS@SharonEstherLampert.com

President of My Fan Club: Rabbi David Posner

Congregation Emanu-El
of the City of New York
Fifth Avenue at Sixty-fifth Street
New York, N.Y. 10021-6595

Study of
DAVID M. POSNER

September 22, 1999

The New York Public Library
Humanities and Social Sciences Library
Fifth Avenue and 42nd Street
New York, NY 10018-2788

Dear Friends:

Sharon Esther Lampert has made application for a fellowship from the Center for Scholars and Writers. It is with greatest pleasure that I write to you in support of her application.

I can best describe this remarkable woman by citing the analysis of Moses Maimonides, in his "Guide for the Perplexed," concerning psychological endowments. He noted the class of people who are intellectually superior, but whose imaginative faculties are deficient. These, he said, were philosophers. Then there are those whose imaginative faculties are highly developed, but who are deficient intellectually. He said these are dreamers and politicians. But then he observed the rare people who have both highly developed intellects and imaginations. These, he said, are prophets.

Sharon Esther Lampert falls into the last category. She has one of the most gifted intellects I have ever encountered, and her imaginative capacity is absolutely awesome.

I have known many people throughout my long career at Temple Emanu-El. I have never met anyone like this extraordinary human being.

Again, awesome is the most appropriate word.

Yours truly,

FORMED BY THE CONSOLIDATION OF EMANU-EL CONGREGATION AND TEMPLE BETH-EL

Sharon Esther Lampert

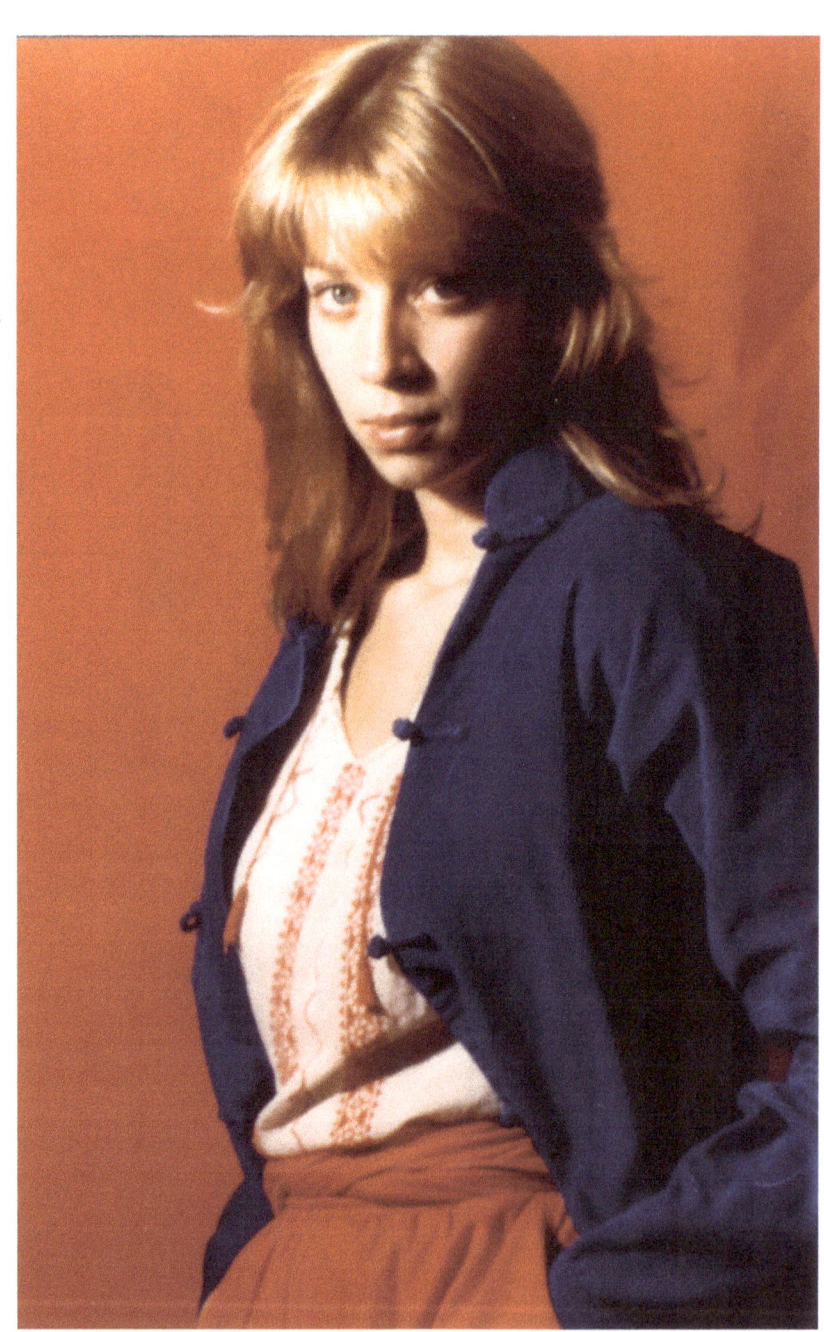

Find The Light and Live In The Light!

Sharon Esther Lampert

Prodigy
Poet
Prophet
Philosopher
Peacemaker
Paladin of Education
PINUP
PHOTON
Player:Jock
Performer
President
Publisher

MYLIFE Is an OPENBOOK, to KNOWME Is to README

God Talks to Me: A Working Definition of God

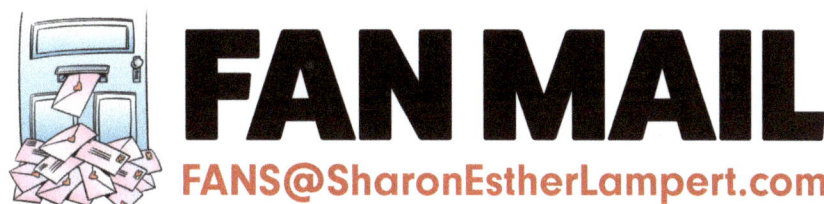

Cody Howell
1042 Prospect Dr.
Imperial, Mo 63052
May 2, 2005

Sharon Esther Lampert
P.O.BOX 103,
New York, New York, 10028, US

Dear, Sharon E. Lampert

Hello, My name in Cody, I am a Junior at Windsor High School in Missouri. I have had the chance to write to any one person and I picked you. I have always enjoyed quotes and sayings. Theirs just something about it, like I have always known there is a "better way" but never really found anything until I started to pay attention that their was more than just physical happenings. The poet has the ability to drink from streams science has yet to discover. I used to always reads one liners like
" a community begins to grow when old men plant trees they know they will never enjoy the shade of." Things like this really interested me. Something more than what I had known.

I am very curious by nature, and this kind of wisdom/intellect really hit the spot for me, now I have many poems, sayings, quotes ext. I can't recite them by heart but I thourouly enjoyed the ones I read. I didn't know of you until me and my buddy were talking about how we like psychology and basically more than average and the "better way". After reading some of your quotes I realized you must have seen your share of happenings and become very wise over the years of thought, poetry, and life.

My first thought was to write to you and try to flatter you because I enjoyed your work. Well I guess you made your poetry your work. Then I started thinking that this well of knowledge, all that stuff you've learned, It would be a long shot but my curiosity wouldn't stop unless if I asked you if you could share some of the knowledge you have gained. Any and all would be appreciated and probably useful later considering I am still just a 17-year-old kid. I can't think of any other word than greedy, but you have already thought so many with your influences, and I ask you to help me out, If your busy you have already done more than enough, thank you, and thanks for your time while reading this. I am sorry but I always find myself looking for more and I'm positive you have gained useful info in your day. I could imagine the child who has heard many stories, lesions, and wisdoms of many. He'd be one of the most diverse ,intelligent humans around, and with something like this in mind how could I not be greedy.

I have already learned some from Internet, friends like the one who told me about poems, and family. I have tried to learn patience from the impatient, kindness from the angry, and truth from fools, but for some reason I'm not thankful for these teachers. I still feel as if I could have more, and the lessons of an older experienced poet just has something about how it sounds. Greatness is all I've seen come from poets their ability to make one think is amazing , I could just imagine the wisdom of an experienced one.

Either way I just wanted to say thank you for your time and thank you for doing what you have done. Your shared wisdom and lessons will help many and your work might not be remembered forever but I believe that your positive effect will. Thank you again

Your student ,
Cody

PINUP
Sharon Esther Lampert

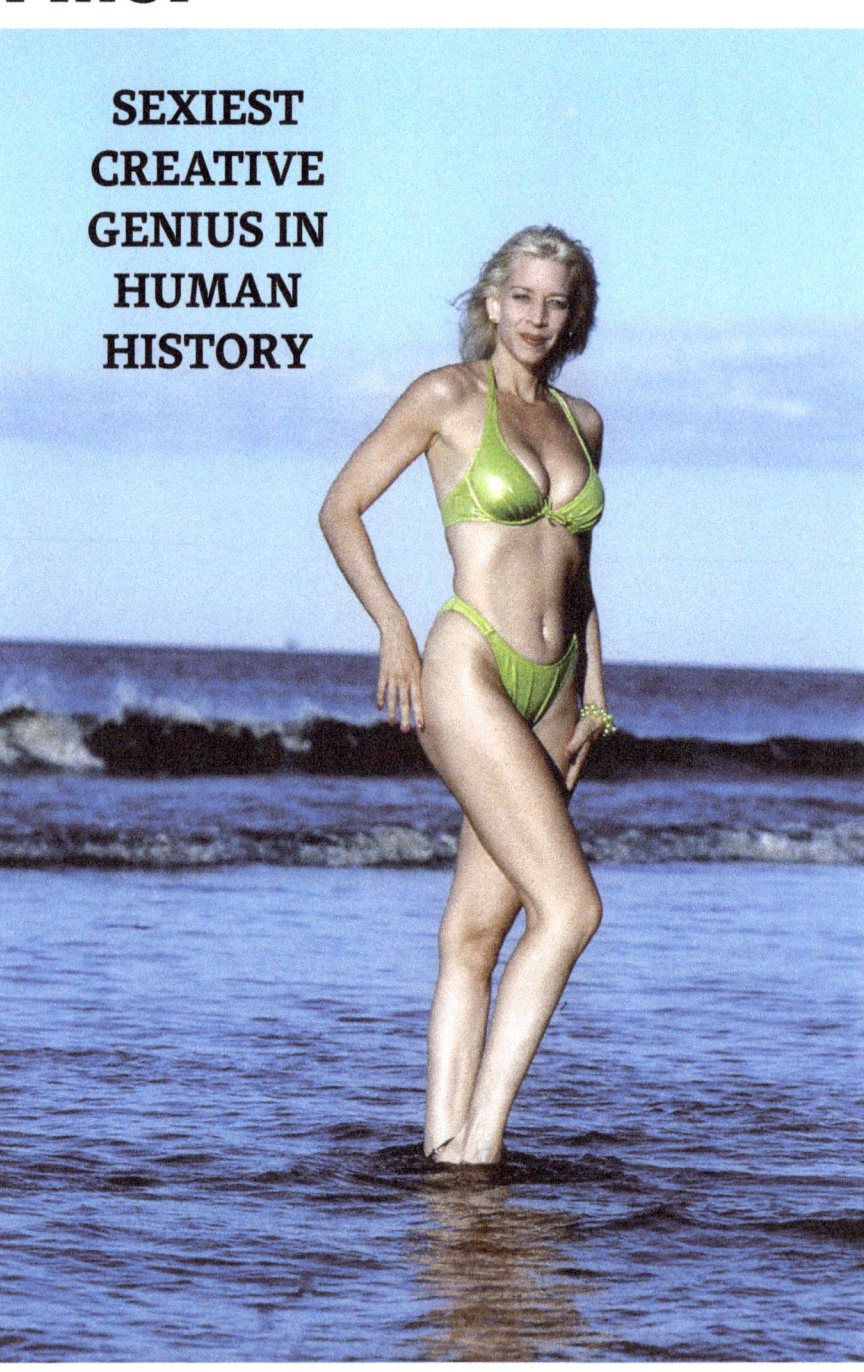

SEXIEST CREATIVE GENIUS IN HUMAN HISTORY

1.
PRODIGY
10 Esoteric Laws of Genius & Creativity

2.
POET
The Greatest Poems Ever Written on Extraordinary World Events

3.
PHILOSOPHER
TEMPORARY INSANITY
Make Life Make Sense
—Written in Letter S

CUPID
Language of Love
—Written in Letter C

4.
PROPHET
22 COMMANDMENTS
A Universal Moral Compass For All People

GOD TALKS TO ME
A WORKING DEFINITION OF GOD
GOD IS GO! DO!

5.
**PHOTON &
PALADIN OF EDUCATION**
SMARTGRADES
BRAIN POWER
REVOLUTION

6.
PINUP
SEXIEST CREATIVE GENIUS IN HUMAN HISTORY

God Talks to Me: A Working Definition of God

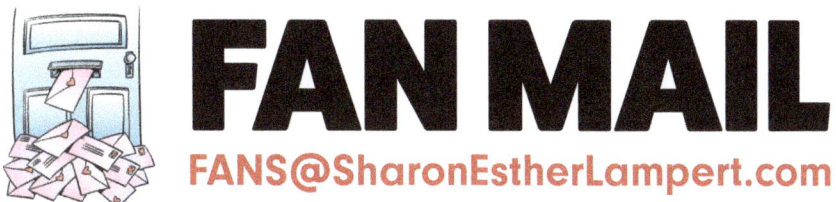

FAN MAIL
FANS@SharonEstherLampert.com

December 2001

Dear Kadimah:
You are truly a remarkable woman. You are a wonderful word-weaver. You are great in spirit and inspire everyone. You have insights on multiple things. You "see" while others stumble along.

That is why you bear the Light. That is why you cry out for Hope in the midst of despair. That is why you are always a step away from the multitude, yet when you speak they cry,

"She is our voice and says what we have felt all the time."

Blessed are those who have you for a friend.
Sincerely,
—Reverend Aaron R. Orr
Hamilton, Ontario, Canada
http://owensinc.freeyellow.com

WHO AM I?
My Name is Aaron Robin Orr and I was born in Belfast, Northern Ireland on November 16, 1940 the only son of Andrew Orr and Hessie Orr. They were Presbyterian by denomination and Christian by life and practice. In September 1965 I married my wife, the former Ruth Hannah Hawkins and never has a man been more blessed than I. We have two children, Elizabeth and Andrew. Beth is married to our son-in-law Remo Pace, gave us our first granddaughter Rachael almost two years ago. Andrew is still single and is involved in various endeavours one of which is writing for an Internet magazine.

SOLVE ONE PROBLEM: EDUCATION: SAVE ENTIRE WORLD

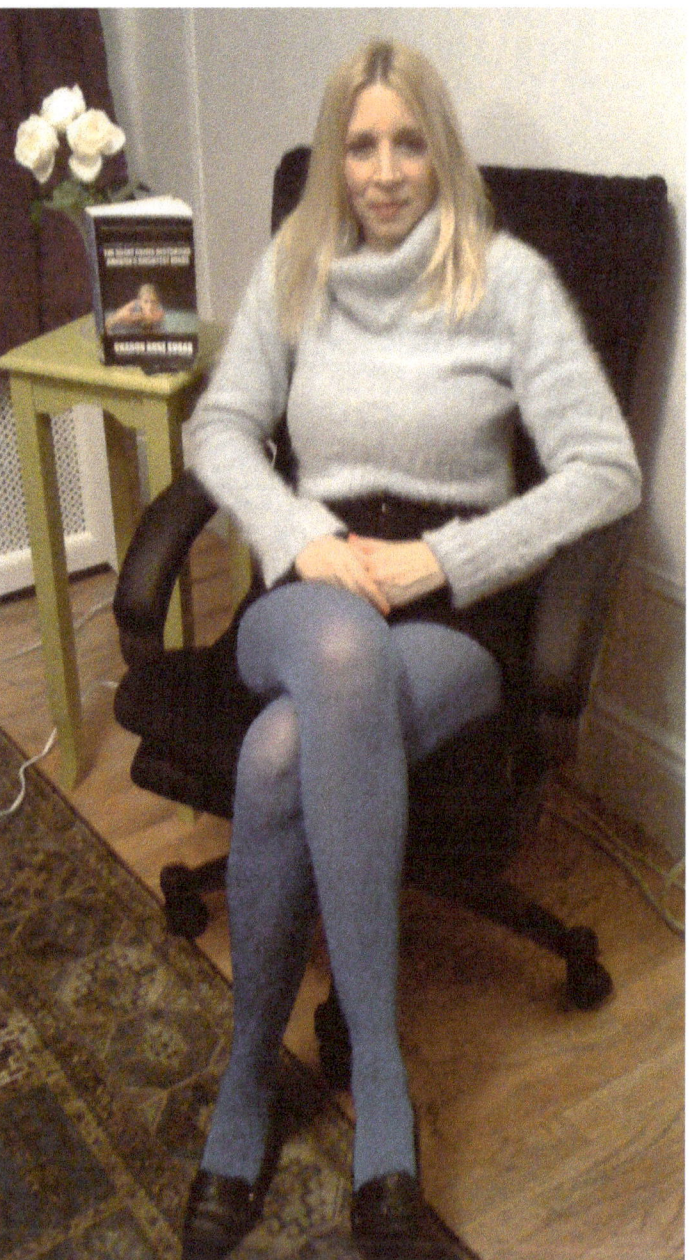

PALADIN OF EDUCATION & PHOTON SUPERHERO

My book was chosen as **BOOK OF THE MONTH** by the Alma Public Library in Wisconsin, **"The Silent Crisis Destroying America's Brightest Minds."** ISBN: 978-1885872548

My Pen Name: Sharon Rose Sugar

SMARTGRADES BRAIN POWER REVOLUTION

Smartgrades.com
EverydayanEasyA.com
BooksNotBombs.com
PhotonSuperHero.com

- The 15 Stepping Stones of Academic Success
- The 15 Stumbling Blocks of Academic Failure
- 10 Learning Tools for Academic Excellence
- 40 Universal Gold Standards of Education
- Parenting for Academic Success

God Talks to Me: A Working Definition of God

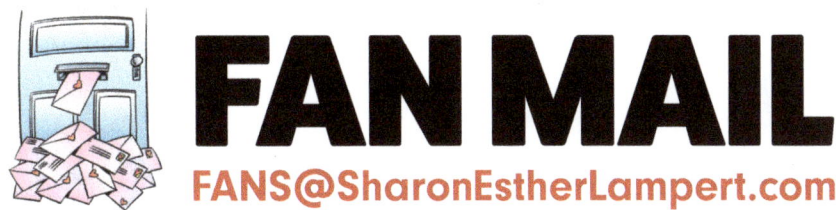

Dear Sharon,

You are not only an exquisite poet, you're beautiful! Am smitten by your luminous beingness. Are you an angel in disguise--a so-called malachim in Hebrew if I am not mistaken.

Thank you for your wonderful open-hearted response. **Your photo will sit next to those of Gautama Buddha and the Blessed Virgin Mary.**

I will follow your sound esoteric advise regarding the positioning of your photo and the two other icons. I am deeply impressed that you are very conscious about the concept of sacred space and the flow of spiritual energy. So please send me your precious photo as soon as possible.

P.S. Will you be generous enough to send me your signed photo which I will place on the secret altar of my heart, lit by the menorah, the seven-stemmed candelabra of your inspiration, O mystical muse, O Rose of Sharon...

Your ardent fan and admirer,
—*Felix Fojas,* **the cybercat with a mystical meow**
Chico, CA, 95926

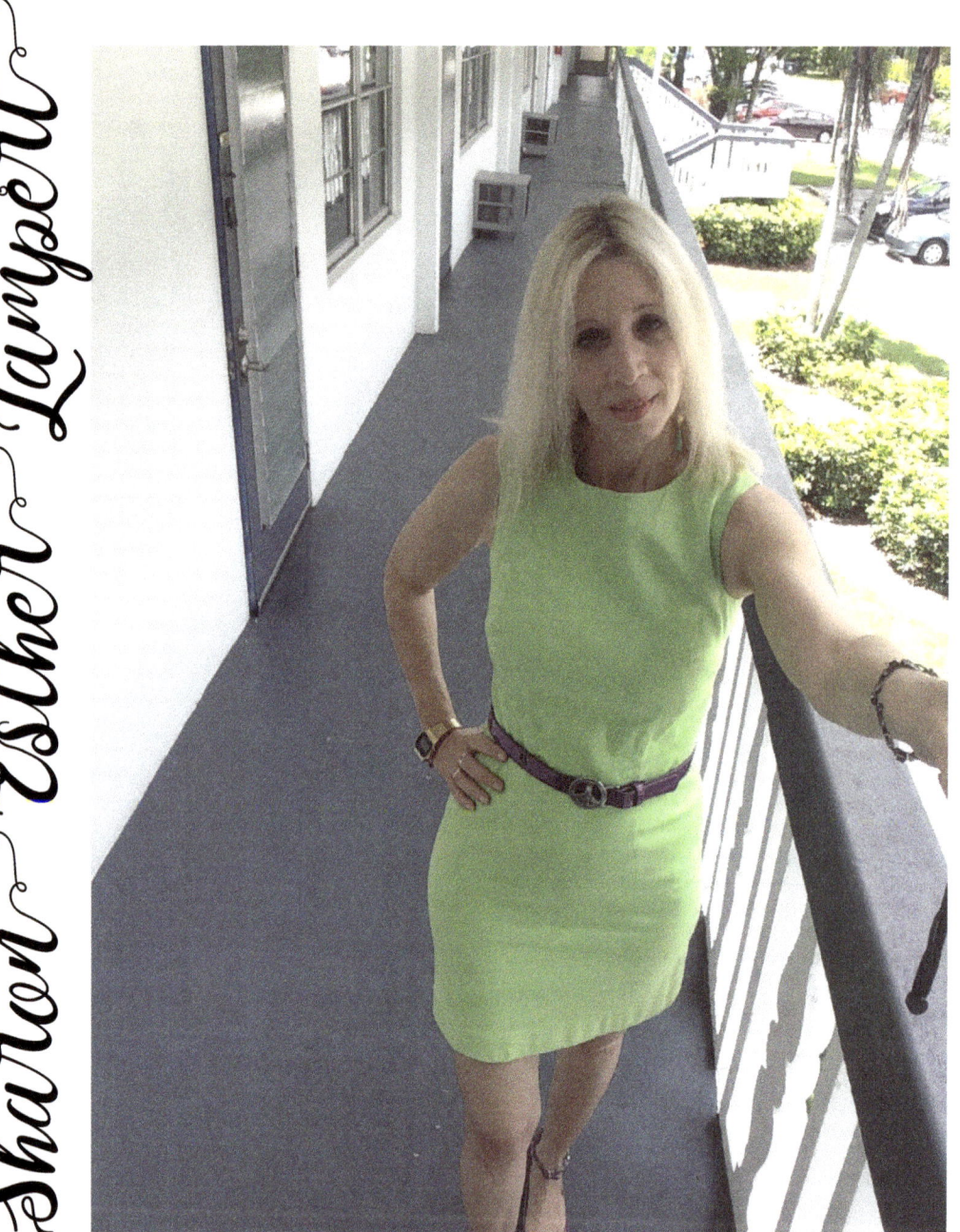

God Talks to Me: A Working Definition of God

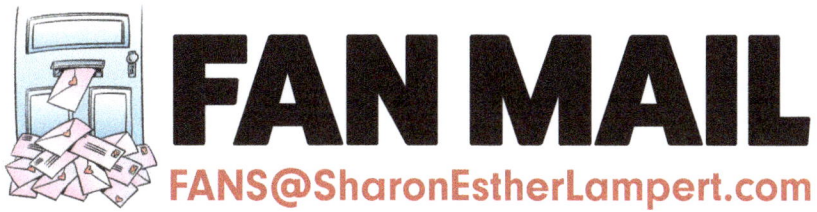

FANS@SharonEstherLampert.com

Dear Sharon,

You are definitely an unusual girl, and what I like is not just your thinking and your brains, but the fact that you are an independent thinker.

People with brains are usually more interesting, but brains aren't a guarantee of that. Sometimes, brains just means they think conventionally, but they do that very well. You don't fit the standard molds.

You have your own style, even in the way you think, it seems. And you are a thorough thinker, and a subtle one, and you are interested in ideas and thinking. I find all that very, VERY attractive, very interesting. It piques my curiosity and I feel like I want to understand more about you and how you think.

Often I get a relatively complete, if rough, "first impression" of people I meet in a fairly short period of contact. With you, after lengthy chat, I couldn't. You are just too complex. Many facets. Very interesting. Certainly an individual. I remember that I liked you very much from our conversation. It was a breath of fresh air, to tell you the truth. I really did enjoy it.

So, if I say "you're a genuine individual, Sharon" I hope it won't sound trite or condescending, because I mean it as a high compliment.

I hope you have friends who understand you, who really understand the parts of you that are most important to you, because you are certainly not cut from any of the "run of the mill" cloths.

I would imagine aesthetics play the major role in photo-selection for a website, but I have to tell you the truth, Sharon: as attractive as the girl on your website is, you are much prettier in person.

Whatever it is, I remember your eyes and your wise, knowing smile and the "kinda sorta" amused, intelligent, perceptive awareness of the world that seemed to be living there behind your expressions, when we were communicating face to face.

— Morry

Artists March to the Beat of a Different Drummer...
Sharon Esther Lampert Marches to the Beat of an Entire Orchestra

Poet, Philosopher, Prophet
Paladin of Education, Peacemaker
Princess & Pea, Phoenix & Prodigy

Princess and the Pea

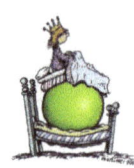

V.E.S.S.E.L.
VERY. EXTRA. SPECIAL.
SHARON. ESTHER. LAMPERT.

Sharon Esther Lampert was born an OLD SOUL — She Was Never Young!

At age nine, her MOMMY declared: "My daughter is a poet, philosopher, and teacher!" She nicknamed her daughter, "The Princess and the Pea!" Sharon's mother was the sole person in Sharon's life who knew who she was from the **INSIDE OUT**! Her mother also knew to her very last breath... the exact day... and to the minute ... when she would die! (Eve Paikoff Lampert: June 3, 1925 — May 5, 1985).

Later in life, Sharon purchased a green-pea pendant, at the Broadway show, "Once Upon a Mattress" starring Sarah Jessica Parker — and wore it every day around her neck with a Jewish star.

Sharon's Gifts Are Metaphysical — Beyond the Scope of Scientific Inquiry

Sharon's greatest literary works woke her up in the middle of the night — and made her get up out of bed — and write them down. There Are No Rough Drafts! — The Books Write Themselves!

On January 31st, 2021, this book was written from 1 p.m. to 10 a.m. One day before, Sharon had no idea she would even write a book! The very next day, lethargy sets in — as being a creative genius is exciting, euphoric, enthralling, enchanting, exhilarating — and exhausting!

The "Princess and the Pea" is a metaphysical phenomemon — inexplicable by scientific inquiry!

When Sharon came home after a day at school, her mother greeted her at the door with the proclaimation:

"The Queen Has Arrived!"

Her father said:

"My Daugher is Fabrent!"
Yiddish: Born with a FIRE is buring under tuchus!   English: Emotionally Intense Disposition

Her brother blurted out:
"My sister is not a normal and regular person — like the rest of us!"

Birth: The Idea of "Sharon" was Conceived in ISRAEL

Her mother was first-generation American, born of Minsk and Pinsk Russian parents; and her father was born in Belarus Russia, and had emmigrated to **Israel**, where they met—but they later married in the USA. Three languages were spoken and sung in Sharon's home: English, Hebrew, and Yiddish.

DNA: Sharon Inherited Two Sets of Artsy-Fartsy Genes

Her father Abraham Lampert was a gifted sculptor, and his nickname was **BEZALEL**, the Biblical artisan who built the **Ark of the Covenant**. Sharon inherited the **BLESSING!** The Museum of Jewish Heritage in NYC featured his Shabbat candlesticks in an exhibit on Cyprus. Her maternal grandfather Benjamin Paikoff was a gifted painter, and made his living as a sign painter of storefronts.

Childhood: Barefoot in a Bikini

Sharon Esther was raised on a beautiful peninsula in Belle Harbor, N.Y., and enjoyed riding the waves of the Atlantic ocean on her raft, barefoot in a bikini — alone and unafraid! Sharon Esther collected sea shells, sea glass and seaweed. Sharon labeled each one with its Latin name — and earned an A grade in Oceanography at Beach Channel High School, Queens, NYC.

Nickname: Daddy Long Legs

Sharon Esther attended the first Robert Gordis Solomon Schecter Conservative Day School, and was the only girl playing soccer on the boys' team. Sharon has very long legs, and was nicknamed, after the spider, **"Daddy Long Legs."** Boys asked to race her in the schoolyard, and no one could catch her, or keep up with her! Even as an adult, Sharon continued to be the only woman who played on men's basketball teams, with men of all different nationalities.

"Faster Than Any Boy, Anywhere, Anytime, Any Age!"
—Sharon Esther Lampert

Fact: There are 5 Books of Moses and 5000 Books of Jewish Comedy!

As a young woman, Sharon proclaimed, "I'm not married, because I have very long legs, and no one was able to catch me!"

As for children, Sharon explained that, "My womb malfunctioned, and I was only able to give birth to kittens: Schmaltzy.com and Falafel!" These cats became internet **SUPERSTARS!** Disarming inquisitive Jewish neighbors with uproarious laughter served her well.

"Keep Them Laughing, Keep Them Sane!"
—Sharon Esther Lampert

"SOLVE ONE PROBLEM: EDUCATION: SAVE THE ENTIRE WORLD!"
—Sharon Esther Lampert

CEO of SMARTGRADES BRAIN POWER REVOLUTION

One of Sharon Esther's outstanding contributions is transforming floundering students into academically successful students. She pioneered the, **SMARTGRADES BRAIN POWER REVOLUTION** learning tools for in-depth comprehension, long-term retention, and mastery of academic material. She documented her case studies in a book titled, **"The Silent Crisis Destroying America's Greatest Minds."** This book was chosen as **Book of the Month** by the Alma Public Library, in Wisconsin, USA. Shop: www.smartgrades.com.

1. Metaphysically Speaking: World Famous Piano Playing Cat MEWOW!

Sharon found a child's toy piano in the garbage — and gave the toy piano to her cat. Her cat started to play the piano, and became a piano virtuoso! Fortunately, cats antics ruled the internet—and Sharon's cats became internet SUPERSTARS. They also have their very own children's book, "SCHMALTZY: In America, Even a Cat Can Have a Dream!" The book has color-coded vocabulary words! You can catch a cat-piano concert on YOUTUBE. Visit: www.schmaltzy.com.

2. Metaphysically Speaking: Poet Hannah Szenes is My Metaphysical Sister

Part 1. At the age of 9, Sharon was cast in a play as Hannah Sezenes, the Hungarian-Israeli poet, who was parachuted into Hungary to save the Jews from the Nazis.

Part 2. Later, Sharon moved to NYC, and found an apartment on the Upper East Side of Manhattan on 82nd Street, that just happened to be situated between the Hungarian Cultural Center and the Hungarian Church; and her best friend Karl Bardosh was a Hungarian Jew, a professor at NYU.

Part 3. Sharon wrote 90% her world famous poems in her cozy-studio apartment.
Later, she successfully rescued his parent's Holocaust documentation—that had been sitting in a drawer for 30 years — and transferred it to the Holocaust museum for safe keeping.

Part 4. Metaphysically speaking: Sharon was parachuted into the middle of the Hungarian community of NYC, and found a Hungarian Jew who needed her help; and rescued Holocaust documentation; and she became a world famous Jewish poet!

Past 5. Sharon was inextricably having an intimate metaphysical relationship with the poet Hannah Szenes that lasted a lifetime. Sharon decided to embrace Hannah Szenzes as family; and every year celebrates her birthday, and remembers her death with birthday and memorial candles.

Hannah had even written a poem about a girl in her dreams who had big-blue eyes! There might be a metaphysical connection here?

3 Degrees from New York University — YOUTUBE Videos

Sharon Esther earned three degrees from NYU, and she was honored with two NYU awards. Sharon represented her class at her graduation — and was honored with an award for "Multi-Interdisciplinary Studies." She also played on the NYU Women's Varsity Basketball Team. Sharon won an NYU Weightlifting Contest — she was the sole contestant — so she won! (Washington Square News article).

"A LIST" Sharon is One of the World's Greatest Poets
#1 Poetry Website for Student Projects

Sharon politely responds to personal, persistent and pesky questions with, "Would you like a gift of poetry?" **Automatic Writing:** All of Sharon's poems are inspired and written in a NY minute.

Sharon never arrives anywhere empty handed, and hands out copies of her poetry to everyone, she meets, and her poetry is greatly appreciated by people from all walks of life.

Never a dull moment, on a NYC public bus, a passenger asks Sharon for all of her pocket poems and handed her pocket poems out to everyone sitting on the bus!

Sharon turns every encounter with a stranger into an ardent fan, and Sharon autographs every poem with her signature gold pen.

On a global scale, Sharon's poetry is used by teachers for their lesson plans, and by students for their school projects.

3. Metaphysically Speaking...
KADIMAH THE 8TH PROPHETESS OF ISRAEL
— THE 22 COMMANDMENTS —
ALL YOU WILL EVER NEED TO KNOW ABOUT GOD

"One afternoon, a flyer from the Kabbalah Center in N.Y.C appeared on my path. I found three flyers that day: on the sidewalk on the way to class, on the bus in the seat next to mine, on the way home — and then a fan emailed me a copy. My gut instinct said that the flyer was talking to me! Its design was similar to a poem I had started — but never finished. I decided to look for that poem; and within a NY minute, **THE 22 COMMANDMENTS** appeared on the page. I made copies to hand out at Chabad Rabbi Krasinofsky's Shabbat luncheon. Right before I handed them out, the Rabbi stood up and said, "Inside every Jewish person is a little Moses trying to get out!" What an introduction! On that note, I handed out **THE 22 COMMANDMENTS.** For years, I read them responsively at a poetry open mic in a Barnes & Noble Bookstore to **RAVE REVIEWS!"** (YOUTUBE video).

Sharon Esther Lampert

THANK YOU
Practice Gratitude — Count Your Blessings

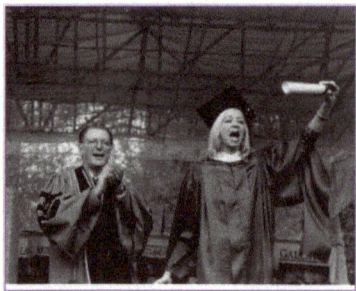
NYU President Jay Oliva and Me

Blessing 1. My Genetics, Two Sets of Artsy-Fartsy Genes and Gift of Genius, Lefty!
- Genetic Inheritance: Painter Maternal Grandfather Benjamin Paikoff & Sculptor Father Abraham Lampert (Exhibit in Museum of Jewish Heritage, NYC)
- Vocalist: Ashira Orchestra, 18 Years: Ramaz Women's Service (YOUTUBE video)
- Athlete: "Faster Than Any Boy, Anytime, Anywhere, Any Age!"

Blessing 2. The Digital Revolution
- **APPLE:** The Golden Age of Personal Computers
- **ADOBE:** The Golden Age of Creativity
- **INGRAM:** The Golden Age of POD Publishing
- **SOCIAL MEDIA:** The Golden Age of Internet & Global Communication
- **iTUNES:** The Golden Age of Music and Lyrics

Blessing 3. My Loved Ones
- **Self-Love:** "**M**indfulness, **M**editation, **M**antra, and **M**usic **M**itigates **MADNESS**!"
- **Unconditional Love:** My **MOMMY** Eve Paikoff Lampert
- My PURRfect Children: SCHMALTZY and FALAFEL (Schmaltzy.com)
- My "Friends First and Forever, and Family" NYU Tisch Professor Karl Bardosh
- My Metaphysical Sister: Poet on a Mission Hannah Sezenes: "**ELI, ELI**"
- My 7 Practice Husbands, Muses, Dates, and NYC Night Life
- My Bubbe Esther Tulkoff (EstherTulkoff.com)

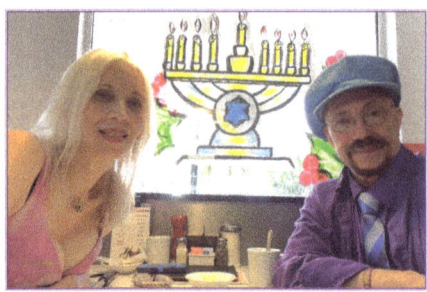
NYU Professor Karl Bardosh and Me

Blessing 4. My NYU Education, Educators, and Awards
My NYU Education: B.A. M.A. M.A. and Awards: (YOUTUBE videos)
- NYU Professor Laurin Raiken NYU "**Multi-Interdisciplinary Award**" and M.A. Class Representative at Graduation
- NYC Rockefeller University, Publication: "Hyperphagia and Obesity Induced by Neuropeptide Y" — Lab of Dr. Sarah Leibowitz and Dr. Glen Stanley
- 100-Year Scholarship Award Winner, Presented by NYC Mayor Edward Koch
- Empire Science Scholarship Award Winner
- Jerusalem Fellowship Award, Aish Hatorah, Israel
- First Prize: Upper East Side Resident Writing Contest
- Voice Teachers: Andy Anselmo of The Singer's Forum, NYC & Estelle Leibling
- Cantor Sherwin Goffin of LSS & Riva Alper of RAMAZ Women's Service (18 Years)

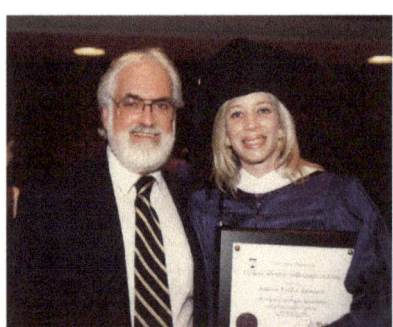
NYU Professor Laurin Raiken and Me

Blessing 5. My Sports
- NYC Marathon
- Basketball: NYU Women's Varsity Basketball Team, Center, NYU Coach Sherri Pickard
- NYU Weightlifting Contest Winner! $16 Million Coles Sports Center (solo contestant — so I won!)
- Basketball: NYC Urban Professional League
- B-Ball Coaches Chicago Bulls Phil Jackson and Boston Celtics Bill Walton
- Basketball and Softball: Coach Sandy Pyonin
- Skiing: Heavenly, Lake Tahoe, Nevada
- Tennis: NYC Central Park Tennis Courts
- Hall of Fame: Wilma Briggs and Jean Harding

Blessing 6. My Inspirations
- **ISRAEL:** "**AM YISRAEL CHAI!**" (Lambs to Slaughter to Lions & Light of the World: **22% Nobel Prizes!**
- **NYC:** The Golden Age of Personal Freedom & Creative Self-Expression
- **AMERICA:** Land of Unlimited Possibility, Potential, and Promise

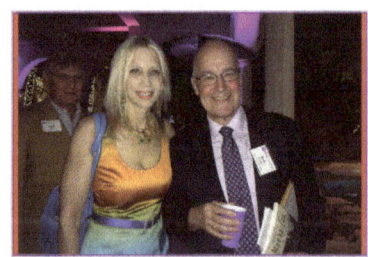
NYU President Andrew Hamilton and Me

God Talks to Me: A Working Definition of God

Teacher Lesson Plan and Student Study Guide

Pick a Question

1. If you could ask God a question — what would it be?
2. Pick 5 of the 32 "Dear God" questions, and answer them from your point of view
3. Write a letter to God, and send it to: DearGod@PhilosopherQueen.com
4. Pick a quote from the list below, and write an English essay

27 Quotes from "God Talks to Me: A Working Definition of God"

1. "GOD IS GO! DO!"
2. "God is Not Physics — The Laws of the Universe! God is Metaphysics — Beyond the Scope of Scientific Inquiry!"
3. "Fight to Live, Live to Fight, Born to Die!"
4. "You Don't Find Love, You Create Love"
5. "Loneliness is Death; Solitude is Divine"
6. "Be Art! You Are Born for Greatness! You Are a Masterpiece!"
7. "Solve One Problem: EDUCATION: Save Entire World!" PHOTON SUPERHERO OF EDUCATION
8. "Meditation, Mindfulness, Mantra and Music Mitigates MADNESS!"
9. "Imperfect World! Imperfect Problem! Imperfect Solution!"
10. "There Are No Believers: There Are Only Make-Believers and Non-Believers! Which One Are You?"
11. "Good People, Nothing is a Problem; Bad People, Everything is a Problem!"
12. "Who Are You? To Ask Me! Who It Is? That I Am!"
13. "Every Day, You Will Be Tested! What Test Did You Take Today?"
14. "Do You Even Exist? Here Today! Gone Tomorrow!"
15. "Dustballs are Domestic Demonic Disturbances!"
16. "Sleep Feels Like I'm Practicing Being Dead!"
17. "Life is Temporary Insanity of Dizzy Daydreams and Crazy Nightmares!"
18. "Find the Light & Live in the Light!"
19. "Women Have All The Power — But Have Never Learned How to Use It!"
20. "You Can Never Know Another Person!"
21. "All People Help You with Their Strengths and Hurt You with Their Weaknesses"
22. "Wherever Jews Go, Grass Grows! Wherever Israelis Go, Gardens Grow!"
23. "The Fine Line Between Genius and Insanity is Organization!"
24. "All Evil is Justified!"
25. "Insanity is the First Law of Nature!"
26. "You Think, Therefore I Am, and God Is!"
27. "We Life Life By Default — Later by Design!"

KADIMAH PRESS: GIFTS OF GENIUS

REVELATION! MY BOOKS WRITE THEMSELVES!

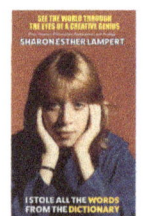

Poet: The Greatest Poems Ever Written on Extraordinary World Events
Title: I Stole All the Words from the Dictionary
ISBN Hardcover: 978-1-885872-06-7
ISBN Paperback: 978-1-885872-07-4
ISBN E-Book: 978-1-885872-08-1

22 Books of Poetry

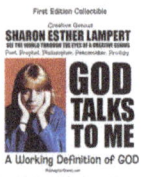

Prophet: WORLD PREMIERE!
Title: God Talks to Me: A Working Definition of God
ISBN Hardcover: 978-1-885872-33-3
ISBN Paperback: 978-1-885872-34-0
ISBN E-Book: 978-1-885872-36-4

40 Books
SMARTGRADES
BRAIN POWER REVOLUTION

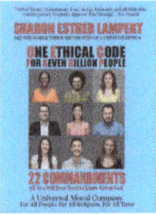

Prophet: WORLD PREMIERE!
A Universal Moral Compass For All Religions, For All People, For All Time
Title: The 22 Commandments: All You Will Ever Need to know About God
ISBN Hardcover: 978-1-885872-03-6
ISBN Paperback: 978-1-885872-04-3
ISBN E-Book: 978-1-885872-05-0

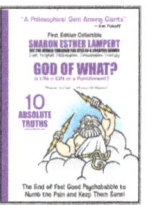

Philosopher: WORLD PREMIERE!
Title: God of What? 11 Esoteric Laws of Inextricability
ISBN Hardcover: 978-1-885872-00-5
ISBN Paperback: 978-1-885872-01-2
ISBN E-Book: 978-1-885872-02-9
Website: GodofWhat.com

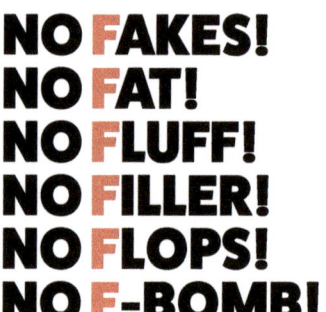

NO **FAKES!**
NO **FAT!**
NO **FLUFF!**
NO **FILLER!**
NO **FLOPS!**
NO **F-BOMB!**

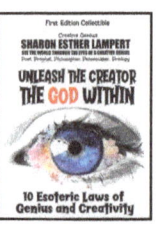

Prodigy: WORLD PREMIERE!
Title: Unleash the Creator The God Within: 10 Esoteric Laws of Genius and Creativity
ISBN Hardcover: 978-1-885872-21-6
ISBN Paperback: 978-1-885872-22-7
ISBN E-Book: 978-1-885872-23-4

God Talks to Me: A Working Definition of God

KADIMAH PRESS: GIFTS OF GENIUS

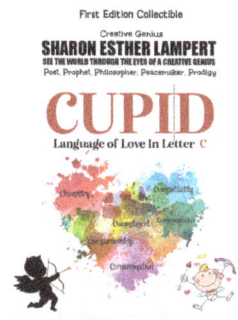

Prodigy: WORLD PREMIERE!
Title: CUPID: Language of Love - Written in Letter C
ISBN Hardcover: 978-1-885872-55-5
ISBN Paperback: 978-1-885872-56-2
ISBN E-Book: 978-1-885872-57-9
Website: SharonEstherLampert.com

MEWOW! PAWTOGRAPHED!

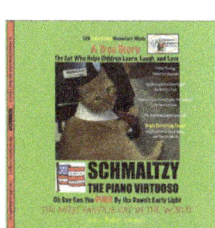

Popular: Children's Book - True Story of a Piano-Playing Cat
Title: SCHMALTZY: In America, Even a Cat Can Have a Dream
ISBN Hardcover: 978-1-885872-39-5
ISBN Paperback: 978-1-885872-38-
ISBN E-Book: 978-1-885872-37-1
Website: Schmaltzy.com

Color-Coded Vocabulary Words Before Every Chaper!

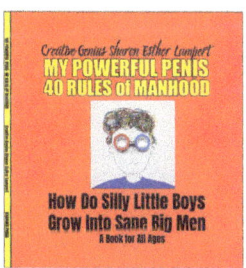

Popular: WORLD PREMIERE!
Title: SILLY LITTLE BOYS: 40 RULES OF MANHOOD
How Do Silly Little Boys Grow into Big Sane Men?
ISBN Hardcover: 978-1-885872-29-6
ISBN Paperback: 978-1-885872-35-7
ISBN E-Book: 978-1-885872-41-8
Website: SillyLittleBoys.com

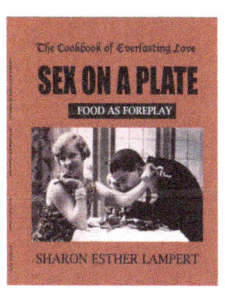

Popular: Every Great Relationship Begins with the Perfect Meal
Title: SEX ON A PLATE: FOOD AS FOREPLAY
The Cookbook of Everlasting Love
ISBN Hardcover: 978-1-885872-46-3
ISBN Paperback: 978-1-885872-48-7
ISBN E-Book: 978-1-885872-47-0
Website: TrueLoveBurnsEternal.com

LITERATURE IS POWERFUL BEYOND WORDS FOR IT CREATES WORLDS

— Sharon Esther Lampert

EVERY THOUGHT IN YOUR HEAD WAS PUT THERE BY A WRITER

— Sharon Esther Lampert

Please Keep in Touch!
Website, Facebook, Twitter, Instagram, YOUTUBE, Pinterest
FANS@SharonEstherLampert.com

God Talks to Me: A *Working* Definition of God

WORLD PEACE EQUATION

The Mathematical and Philosophical Proof for World Peace

$$VG + VL = VP$$

Virtue of the Good + Value of Life = Vision of Peace

$$VG+VL=VP$$
$$VP=VG+VL$$
$$VP=V(G+L)$$
$$P=(G+L)$$

Peace = Good + Life

Peace = Good Life

Sharon Esther Lampert
Princess Kadimah 8TH Prophetess of Israel
Gift Shop: WorldPeaceEquation.com

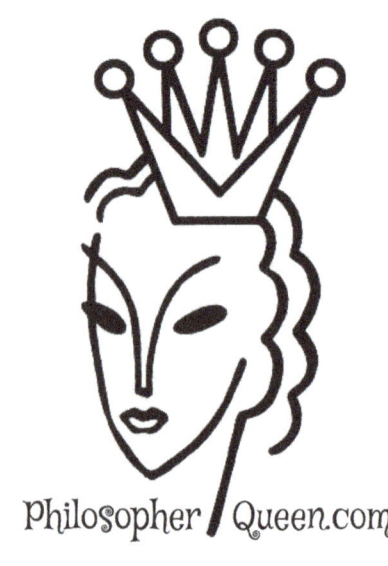

It is always good to hear from you!
DearGod@PhilosopherQueen.com
Go to Work! Writing is Rewriting!

GOD IS GO! DO!

I Am Mortal.
My Books Are Immortal.
My Books Are My Remains.
Please Handle Them Gently.

REVELATION: THE BOOK THAT WROTE ITSELF

January 31, 2021, 1 a.m. — 10 a.m.

Sharon Esther Lampert
SEE THE WORLD THORUGH THE EYES OF A CREATIVE GENIUS
Prophet, Poet, Philosopher, Peacemaker, Princess & Pea, and Prodigy

FANS@SharonEstherLampert.com

Your work is going to fill a large part of your life, and the only way to be truly satisfied is to do what you believe is great work. And the only way to do great work is to love what you do. If you haven't found it yet, keep looking. Don't settle. As with all matters of the heart, you'll know when you find it.

—Steve Jobs, APPLE

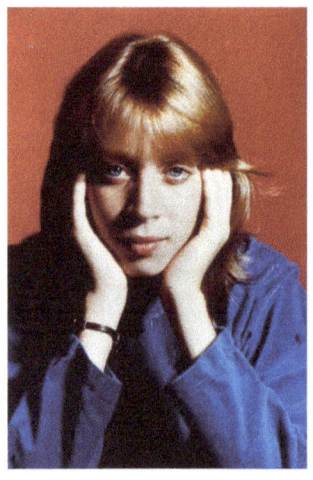

Ask God a Question:
Prophet@GodIsGoDo.com

I am a prophet.
I deliver the message.
What you do with the message is your business!

Prophetess Sharon Esther Lampert

SEE THE WORLD THORUGH THE EYES OF A CREATIVE GENIUS
Prophet, Poet, Philosopher, Peacemaker, Princess & Pea, and Prodigy

Four Books with God in the Title:

* Who Knew God Was Such a Chattrbox
* The 22 Commandments: All You Will Ever Need to Know About God
* 10 Esoteric Laws of Genius & Inextricability: Unleash the Creator The God With Within
* God of What? 11 Esoteric Laws of Inextricability

www.ingramcontent.com/pod-product-compliance
Lightning Source LLC
Chambersburg PA
CBHW042354280426
43661CB00095B/1042